Hemodynamic Waveforms
Exercises in Identification and Analysis

To the
critical care specialists
who provide the essential link in patient care
in coronary care units and intensive care units
throughout the world

Hemodynamic Waveforms
Exercises in Identification and Analysis

ELAINE KIESS DAILY, RN, BS, RCVT
Clinical Cardiovascular Research Nurse
University of California-San Diego Medical Center
San Diego, California

with the assistance of
JOHN SPEER SCHROEDER, MD
Professor of Medicine (Cardiology)
Cardiology Division, Department of Medicine
Stanford University School of Medicine
Stanford, California

SECOND EDITION

with 179 illustrations

The C. V. Mosby Company
St. Louis • Baltimore • Philadelphia • Toronto   1990

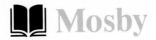

Executive Editor: Don Ladig
Developmental Editor: Jeanne Rowland
Project Manager: Patricia Tannian
Production Editor: Teresa Breckwoldt
Designer: Susan E. Lane

SECOND EDITION

Printed in the United States of America

The C.V. Mosby Company
11830 Westline Industrial Drive, St. Louis, Missouri 63146

Library of Congress Cataloging in Publication Data

Daily, Elaine Kiess.
    Hemodynamic waveforms : exercises in identification and analysis /
Elaine Kiess Daily, John Speer Schroeder. — 2nd ed.
        p.   cm.
    Includes bibliographical references.
    ISBN 0-8016-6141-2
    1.   Hemodynamic monitoring—Problems, exercises, etc.
2. Cardiovascular system—Diseases—Nursing.   I.   Schroeder, John
Speer, 1937-   . II.   Title.
    [DNLM: 1.   Electrocardiography—nurses' instruction.
2. Hemodynamics—nurses' instruction.   3.   Monitoring, Physiologic—
nurses' instruction.   WG   106   D133h]
RC670.5.H45D34   1990
616.07'54—dc20
DNLM/DLC
for Library of Congress   90-5482
                                                                                      CIP

GW/VH/VH   9   8   7   6   5   4   3   2   1

Preface

Our experience lecturing to critical care nurses and specialists throughout the United States has made us acutely aware of the need for practical experience in identifying and interpreting hemodynamic waveforms. Thus the purpose of this book is to provide this experience by presenting the opportunity to study a variety of hemodynamic pressure waveforms. It is hoped that this book will serve as a detailed supplement to our *Techniques in Bedside Hemodynamic Monitoring,* ed. 6 (1989, The CV Mosby Co.), which provides basic discussion, information, guidelines, and techniques. This book is intended for the individual who has a solid foundation in the physiology and techniques of hemodynamic monitoring and who is now ready for more intense, practical learning experiences. Those pressure waveforms that appear in *Techniques in Bedside Hemodynamic Monitoring,* ed. 6, are primarily ideal, normal tracings selected to teach the physiologic events responsible for the pressure changes. Unfortunately, the ideal, normal pressure tracing is seldom encountered in the clinical situation. Although they are necessary and useful to teach the basic principles of hemodynamic monitoring, they are not always practical. This book, then, expands on the reader's basic knowledge and offers a variety of actual pressure tracings of the type encountered in the clinical setting.

The first five chapters review the physiologic events that produce specific hemodynamic waveforms, as well as their correlation to the ECG and causes of commonly seen abnormalities. Following the discussions are examples of numerous, varied, normal and abnormal hemodynamic waveforms with analysis and pertinent comments. Chapter 6 includes case studies of individual patients to illustrate the hemodynamic abnormalities in certain disorders. The last chapter is a self-assessment section in which the reader can exercise skills in identification and analysis of various hemodynamic waveforms. One correct interpretation is on the reverse side of the page for immediate reinforcement or correction. Many of the hemodynamic waveforms throughout this book could be due to more than one pathologic condition. To enhance learning and avoid the confusion of a long list of possible causes, we have listed only the most likely pathologic condition. Needless to say, the experienced hemodynamicist could determine other, equally correct causes of the abnormality.

We hope that use of this book will lead to a greater understanding of the physiologic causes of hemodynamic pressure waveforms, improve identification and interpretation skills, and thereby ease the problems that all too often are associated with hemodynamic monitoring.

Slide series

In response to the numerous requests we have had for duplications of the waveform illustrations in this book, we have compiled a series of slides representing all the hemodynamic waveforms in this book. Each slide is numbered to correspond to the appropriate page number of this book. We hope this slide series will serve as a valuable educational tool when used in conjunction with the text of this book. We anticipate its being particularly useful for hospital in-service, private, and institutional educational programs in cardiovascular medicine and hemodynamic monitoring. This slide series may be obtained by completing the order form on the last page of this book.

Our goal remains to meet the learning needs of health personnel involved in hemodynamic monitoring by providing enhanced educational material.

ELAINE KIESS DAILY
JOHN SPEER SCHROEDER

Contents

Hemodynamic Waveforms
Exercises in Identification and Analysis

Chapter 1

Right Atrial Pressures

Physiology and Morphology

The pressure changes produced by the right atrium are small and usually consist of three distinct positive waves—a, c, and v—followed by negative waves—x, x^1, and y descents. The a wave is a small pressure rise that is produced by the action of atrial systole. The decline in pressure that immediately follows the a wave is termed the x descent and reflects atrial relaxation (immediately following systole). The c wave may appear as a distinct wave, as a notch on the downslope of the a wave, the upslope of the v wave, or may be absent altogether. It reflects a slight increase in pressure in the right atrium produced by closure of the tricuspid valve leaflets. The negative wave immediately following the c wave is termed the x^1 descent. It is produced by a downward pulling of the septum during ventricular systole. (If the c wave appears only as notch on the a wave, the single descent following the ac wave is termed the x descent.)

The v wave is an increase in atrial pressure produced by right atrial filling during concomitant right ventricular systole, which causes the leaflets of the closed tricuspid valve to actually bulge back into the right atrium. The y descent immediately follows the v wave and is produced by the opening of the tricuspid valve and emptying of the right atrium into the right ventricle.

Since the pressure rises produced during both the atrial systolic (a wave) and diastolic (v wave) events are nearly the same (usually within 3 to 4 mm Hg of each other), we generally take an average or a mean of the pressure rises. The normal resting mean right atrial pressure is 2 to 6 mm Hg.

Normal variations during spontaneous respiration include a decline in the right atrial (RA) pressure during spontaneous inhalation as intrathoracic pressure becomes more negative, and a rise in pressure during exhalation. The opposite effect is seen when patients are mechanically ventilated. More accurate hemodynamic pressure readings are obtained when measured at end-expiration at which time intrathoracic pressure changes are minimal. This usually requires the use of a graphic recording of the waveform to discern end-expiration.

ECG Correlation

The a wave, which represents mechanical atrial systole, immediately succeeds electrical atrial depolarization, that is, after the P wave of the ECG. Because of the time required for the mechanical event to reach the sensing device (the transducer) and depending on the length of tubing used, there is a varying degree of delay between the recorded electrical event and the mechanical event. At any rate, the *a* wave of the atrial pressure generally is seen 80 to 100 msecs after the P wave or at some time within the PR interval of the ECG.

The *c* wave, reflecting closure of the tricuspid valve, corresponds to the RS-T junction of the ECG. Its timing following the *a* wave approximates the PR interval.

The *v* wave, occurring during ventricular systole, succeeds electrical ventricular depolarization and can be looked for at the end of the electrocardiographic T wave or any time in the TP interval.

Atrial fibrillation is characterized by the absence of uniform atrial depolarization and consequently results in absent P waves in the ECG and therefore absent *a* waves in the right atrial pressure waveform. Following each T wave one distinct pressure rise, the *v* wave, occurs. Frequently, however, it is possible to see small flutter or fibrillatory waves throughout the pressure tracing. The presence of regular, distinct flutter waves in the RA waveform can be seen in patients with atrial flutter. Identification of these waveforms is easiest if the monitor sweep or paper recording speed is increased (see Figure 1-8).

In *junctional rhythm* or during certain beats of *AV dissociation* where the atria contract against a closed tricuspid valve, giant *a* or cannon *a* waves are seen in the RA pressure tracing. Cannon *a* waves also can be seen following a premature ventricular contraction (PVC) and irregularly during ventricular tachycardia. Again, reviewing the ECG and the atrial waveform at faster paper speed (50 mm/sec) facilitates correct identification.

Patients with a ventricular pacemaker may have absent *a* waves, occasional, random *a* waves, or even cannon *a* waves at times depending on the underlying rhythm. This is the result of absent or dissociated atrial activity that does not relate to the QRS.

Abnormal Findings

Elevated RA pressures occur in the following cases:
1. Right ventricular failure
2. Tricuspid stenosis and regurgitation
3. Cardiac tamponade
4. Constrictive pericarditis
5. Pulmonary hypertension (primary or secondary)
6. Chronic left ventricular failure
7. Volume overload

The *a* wave of the RA pressure tracing is exaggerated and elevated in any condition that increases the resistance to right ventricular filling. These include tricuspid stenosis, RV failure, pulmonary hypertension, and pulmonic stenosis (Figure 1-8).

The *v* wave of the RA pressure tracing is exaggerated and elevated in tricuspid regurgitation as a result of a reflux of blood into the right atrium during ventricular systole through the insufficiently closed tricuspid valve (Figure 1-12). Generally, the *y* descent following the *v* wave is steeper, reflecting increased volume changes as the normal RA volume plus the regurgitant volume exit the right atrium to fill the right ventricle. Clinically, tricuspid regurgitation most commonly occurs as a result of acute RV failure and dilatation.

In cardiac tamponade both the *a* and *v* waves are equally elevated and reflect the elevated diastolic filling pressures in all chambers of the heart. The contour of the RA pressure tracing is distinct, however, showing a predominant *x* descent with a very short or absent *y* descent (Figure 1-8). The *y* descent becomes attenuated or almost absent as a result of diminished volume exiting the right atrium to fill the right ventricle. The mean value of the RA pressure becomes elevated and equals or approximates the mean pulmonary artery wedge (PAW) and pulmonary artery (PA) end-diastolic values.

In constrictive pericardial disease the *a* and *v* waves of the RA pressure tracing are also elevated, but the contour of the waveform differs from that of cardiac tamponade, showing either a brief or normal *x* descent with a predominant *y* descent, or equally dominant *x* and *y* descents (Figure 1-11). The exaggerated *y* descent is a result of rapid ventricular filling (atrial emptying) during early diastole followed by an abrupt rise in pressure as the size of the heart is increased and compressed by the inelastic, constricted pericardium. Additionally, Kussmaul's sign (a rise rather than a fall in right atrial pressure during inspiration) can be seen in constrictive disease but rarely, if ever, in cardiac tamponade.

Kussmaul's sign and elevation of the RA waveform with an *xY* or *xy* pattern also can be seen in patients with acute RV infarction in which an acutely dilated right ventricle is restricted by the noncompliant pericardium.

As in cardiac tamponade, the value of the mean RA pressure in constrictive pericarditis usually equals both the PAW and PA end-diastolic pressures.

↑ A$_w$: ↑S, RVF, PHTN, PS

↑ V$_w$: ↑R

A & V$_w$ ↑: C. tamponade ;→ predominant x descend c̄ Short or Ø Y desc (X$_{ys}$)

Constrictive P: A & V$_w$ are Elevated, → brief or NL x desc c̄ Predominant Y descent (xY)

Kussmauls Sign: ⊕ in Constric Disea
ie: a Rise (not fall) during insp in RA

RVMI: ↑A, V$_w$, xY or xy Config

EXAMPLES

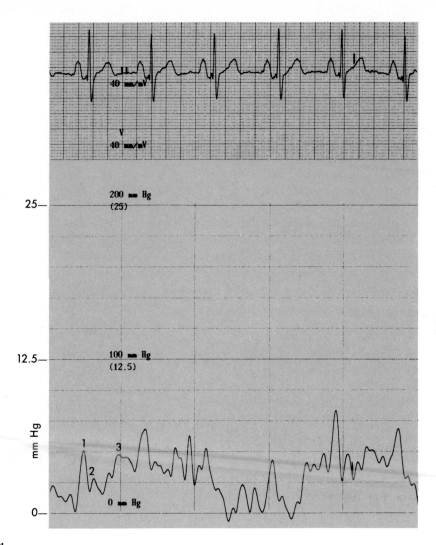

FIGURE 1-1

ANALYSIS

Rhythm: NSR

Pressure(s): RA

Waveform characteristics and measurements:

1.	*a* Wave	; 5	mm Hg
2.	*c* Wave	;	mm Hg
3.	*v* Wave	; 4	mm Hg
4.	Mean	; 4	mm Hg
5.		;	mm Hg
6.		;	mm Hg
7.		;	mm Hg

Suspected abnormality/diagnosis: Normal right heart pressure

Comments: Normal RA contour and pressure with appropriate respiratory variation.

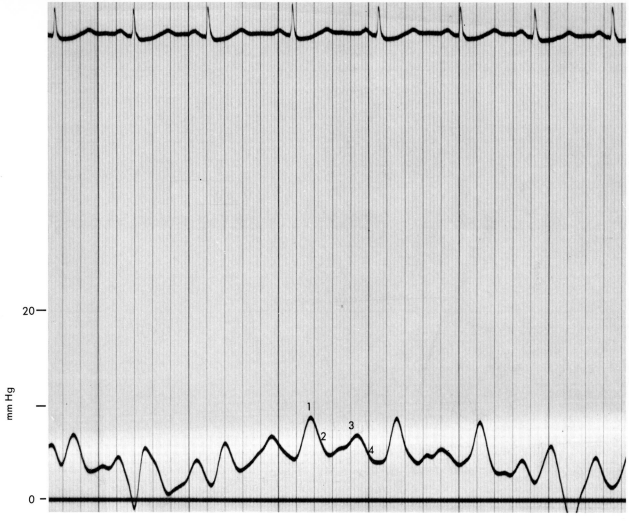

FIGURE 1-2

ANALYSIS

Rhythm: NSR

Pressure(s): RA

Waveform characteristics and measurements:

1.	*a* Wave	;	7	mm Hg
2.	*x* Descent	;		mm Hg
3.	*v* Wave	;	6	mm Hg
4.	*y* Descent	;		mm Hg
5.	Mean	;	5	mm Hg
6.		;		mm Hg
7.		;		mm Hg

Suspected abnormality/diagnosis: Normal

Comments: Note the normal respiratory variation with a fall in atrial pressure during inspiration.

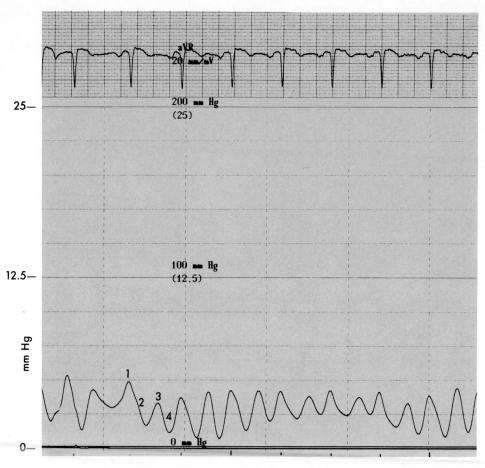

FIGURE 1-3

ANALYSIS

Rhythm: NSR

Pressure(s): RA

Waveform characteristics and measurements:

1.	*a* Wave	;	4	mm Hg
2.	*x* Descent	;		mm Hg
3.	*v* Wave	;	4	mm Hg
4.	*y* Descent	;		mm Hg
5.	Mean	;	4	mm Hg
6.		;		mm Hg
7.		;		mm Hg

Suspected abnormality/diagnosis: Normal right heart filling pressures

Comments:

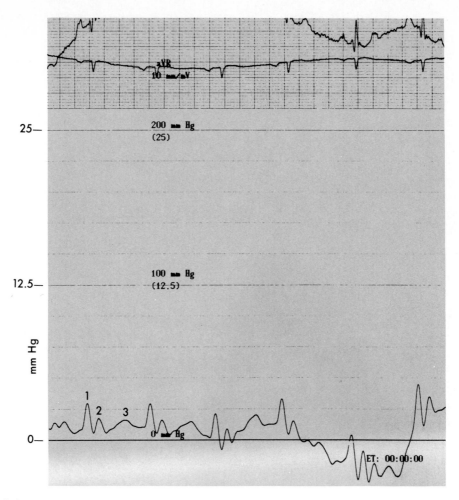

FIGURE 1-4

ANALYSIS

Rhythm: NSR

Pressure(s): RA

Waveform characteristics and measurements:

1.	*a* Wave	;	1	mm Hg
2.	*c* Wave	;		mm Hg
3.	*v* Wave	;	1	mm Hg
4.	Mean	;	1	mm Hg
5.		;		mm Hg
6.		;		mm Hg
7.		;		mm Hg

Suspected abnormality/diagnosis: Normal or hypovolemia

Comments: In conjunction with an adequate stroke volume and cardiac output, this low RA pressure would be considered normal, but if associated with any evidence of hypoperfusion, such as low right heart preload, it would indicate hypovolemia.

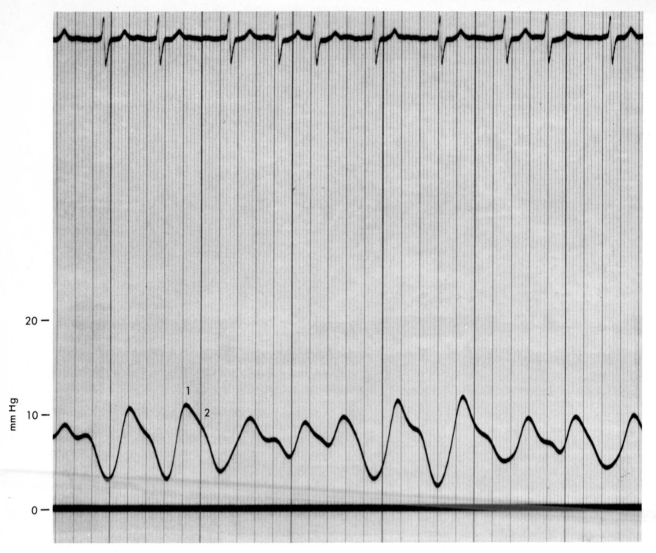

FIGURE 1-5

ANALYSIS

Rhythm: Atrial fibrillation

Pressure(s): RA

Waveform characteristics and measurements:

1.	v Wave	;	10	mm Hg
2.	y Descent	;		mm Hg
3.	Mean	;	8	mm Hg
4.		;		mm Hg
5.		;		mm Hg
6.		;		mm Hg
7.		;		mm Hg

Suspected abnormality/diagnosis: Mild RV failure

Comments: Note the effect of changing RR intervals on the extent of the y descent reflecting changes in duration of RV filling. The absence of an a wave is due to atrial fibrillation.

8

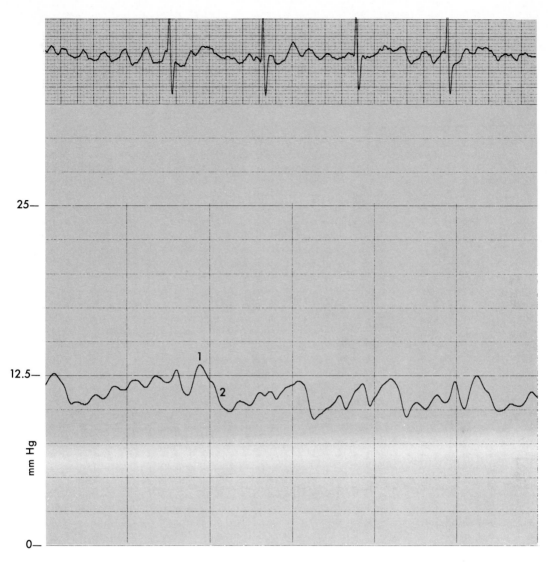

FIGURE 1-6

ANALYSIS

Rhythm: Atrial fibrillation/flutter

Pressure(s): RA

Waveform characteristics and measurements:

1.	*a* Wave	;	mm Hg
2.	*y* Descent	;	mm Hg
3.	Mean	; 11	mm Hg
4.		;	mm Hg
5.		;	mm Hg
6.		;	mm Hg
7.		;	mm Hg

Suspected abnormality/diagnosis: Mild right heart failure

Comments: This RA pressure is elevated with obvious flutter waves apparent in the waveform.

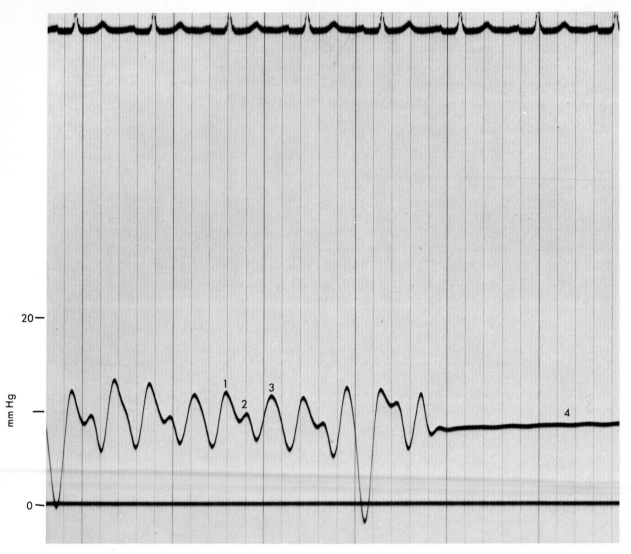

FIGURE 1-7

ANALYSIS

Rhythm: NSR with prolonged PR interval

Pressure(s): RA

Waveform characteristics and measurements:

1.	*a* Wave	;	14	mm Hg
2.	*c* Wave	;		mm Hg
3.	*v* Wave	;	14	mm Hg
4.	Electrical mean	;	10	mm Hg
5.		;		mm Hg
6.		;		mm Hg
7.		;		mm Hg

Suspected abnormality/diagnosis: Hypervolemia or RV failure

Comments: Note exaggerated inspiratory response bringing the *y* descent below baseline at times, and the clearly defined *c* wave that becomes more evident with increases in the PR interval.

10

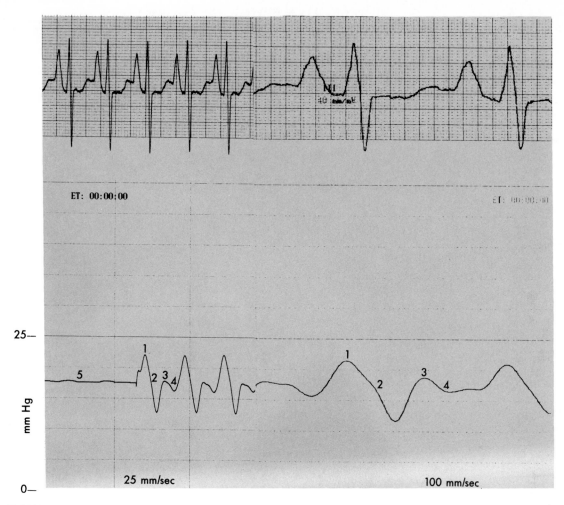

ET: 00:00:00

ET: 00:00:00

25—

mm Hg

0—

25 mm/sec

100 mm/sec

FIGURE 1-8

ANALYSIS

Rhythm: NSR

Pressure(s): RA

Waveform characteristics and measurements:

1.	*a* Wave	; 22	mm Hg
2.	*x* Descent	;	mm Hg
3.	*v* Wave	; 17	mm Hg
4.	*y* Descent	;	mm Hg
5.	Mean	; 17	mm Hg
6.		;	mm Hg
7.		;	mm Hg

Suspected abnormality/diagnosis: Right heart failure

Comments: The dominant and elevated *a* wave of this RA pressure indicates right heart failure with increased resistance to ventricular filling. Increasing the paper speed from 25 mm/sec to 100 mm/sec facilitates accurate identification of the waveform components.

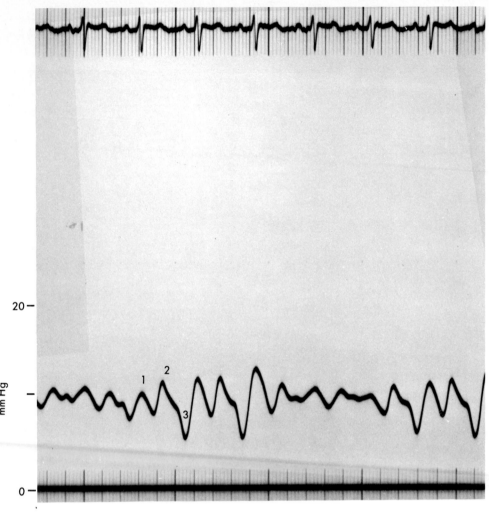

FIGURE 1-9

ANALYSIS

Rhythm: NSR

Pressure(s): RA

Waveform characteristics and measurements:

1.	*a* Wave	; 11	mm Hg
2.	*v* Wave	; 12	mm Hg
3.	*y* Descent	;	mm Hg
4.		;	mm Hg
5.		;	mm Hg
6.		;	mm Hg
7.		;	mm Hg

Suspected abnormality/diagnosis: Mild RV failure

Comments: Moderately elevated *a* and *v* waves in a patient with mild RV failure.

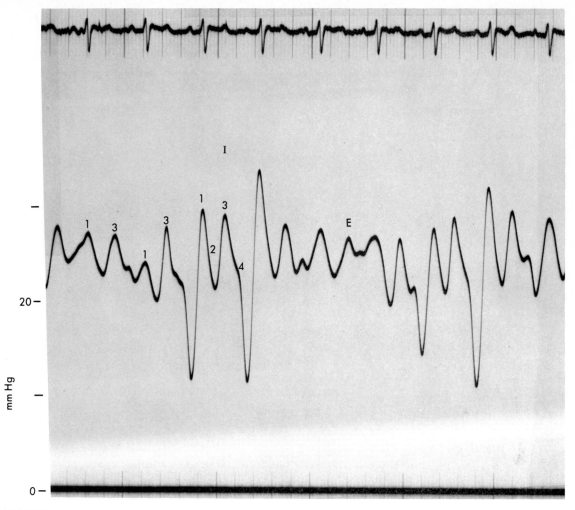

FIGURE 1-10

ANALYSIS

Rhythm: NSR

Pressure(s): RA

Waveform characteristics and measurements:

1.	*a* Wave	;	28	mm Hg
2.	*x* Descent	;		mm Hg
3.	*v* Wave	;	27	mm Hg
4.	*y* Descent	;		mm Hg
5.	Mean	;	25	mm Hg
6.		;		mm Hg
7.		;		mm Hg

Suspected abnormality/diagnosis: RV failure possibly secondary to RV infarction

Comments: Note the marked respiratory variation with exaggeration of the *y* descent and increase in pressure during inspiration (Kussmaul's sign). This is a common finding in patients with acute RV infarction.

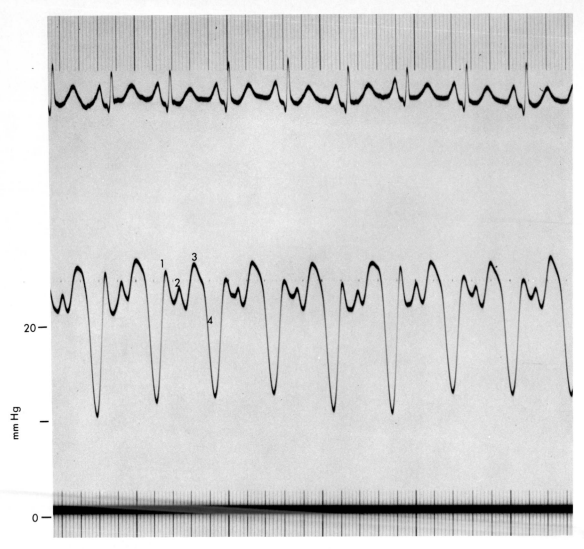

FIGURE 1-11

ANALYSIS

Rhythm: NSR

Pressure(s): RA

Waveform characteristics and measurements:

1.	*a* Wave	;	25	mm Hg
2.	*c* Wave	;		mm Hg
3.	*v* Wave	;	27	mm Hg
4.	*y* Descent	;		mm Hg
5.	Mean	;	19	mm Hg
6.		;		mm Hg
7.		;		mm Hg

Suspected abnormality/diagnosis: Constrictive pericarditis

Comments: Note the elevated *a* and *v* waves with an exaggerated *y* descent consistent with constrictive pericardial disease. The exaggerated *y* descent is due to rapid ventricular filling (atrial emptying) during early diastole followed by an abrupt rise in pressure as the size of the heart is increased and compressed by the inelastic, constricted pericardium.

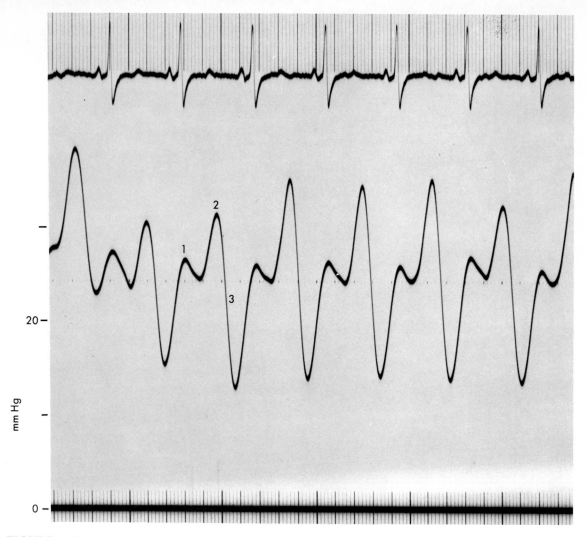

FIGURE 1-12

ANALYSIS

Rhythm: NSR

Pressure(s): RA

Waveform characteristics and measurements:

1.	*a* Wave	;	26	mm Hg
2.	*v* Wave	;	34	mm Hg
3.	*y* Descent	;		mm Hg
4.		;		mm Hg
5.		;		mm Hg
6.		;		mm Hg
7.		;		mm Hg

Suspected abnormality/diagnosis: RV Failure with tricuspid insufficiency secondary to RV infarction

Comments: Both the *a* and *v* waves of this RA waveform are elevated; however, the *v* wave is dominant followed by a rapid *y* descent. This is due to tricuspid regurgitation with an increase in blood volume in the right atrium during ventricular systole. The *a* wave of 26 mm Hg reflects an elevated RVedp and RV failure. This type of hemodynamic picture can be seen in RV infarction, with dilatation of the right ventricle producing functional tricuspid regurgitation.

15

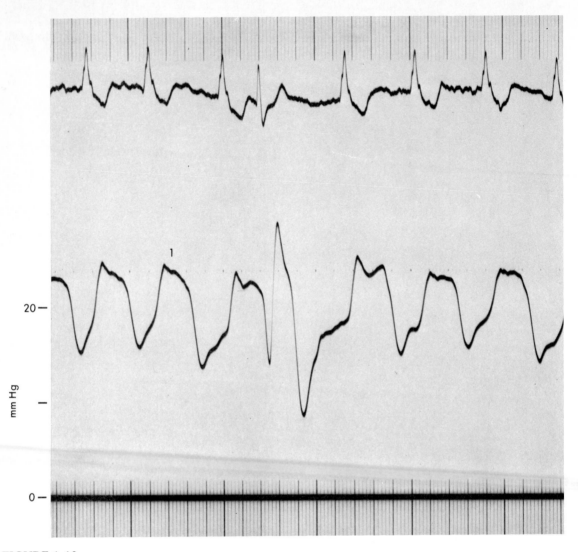

FIGURE 1-13

ANALYSIS

Rhythm: Atrial fibrillation with PNB

Pressure(s): RA

Waveform characteristics and measurements:

1.	v Wave	;	24	mm Hg
2.	Mean	;	18	mm Hg
3.		;		mm Hg
4.		;		mm Hg
5.		;		mm Hg
6.		;		mm Hg
7.		;		mm Hg

Suspected abnormality/diagnosis: RV failure with tricuspid regurgitation secondary to RV dilatation

Comments: Note the increased v wave following the premature nodal beat.

16

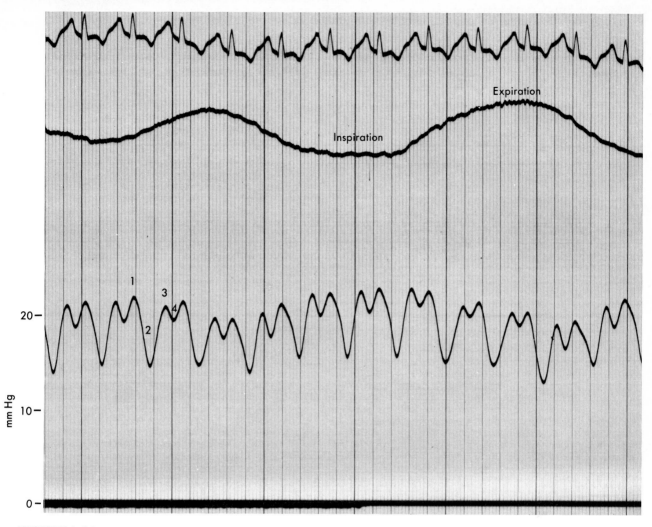

20 —

10 —

0 —

mm Hg

Inspiration

Expiration

1
2
3
4

FIGURE 1-14

ANALYSIS

Rhythm: Sinus tachycardia

Pressure(s): RA

Waveform characteristics and measurements:

1.	*a* Wave	;	20	mm Hg
2.	*x* Descent	;		mm Hg
3.	*v* Wave	;	20	mm Hg
4.	*y* Descent	;		mm Hg
5.	Mean	;	19	mm Hg
6.		;		mm Hg
7.		;		mm Hg

Suspected abnormality/diagnosis: Effusive-constrictive pericardial disease

Comments: Effusive-constrictive pericarditis refers to a combined condition in which there is both visceral pericardial constriction and the presence of effusion in the pericardial space. The RA pressure is elevated as a compensatory mechanism to adequately fill the heart. The contour of the RA pressure usually discloses approximately equal *a* and *v* waves with either a prominent *x* descent (as in cardiac tamponade) or equal *x* and *y* descents. Normally the atrial pressure falls during inspiration due to negative intrathoracic pressure. Note the rise, rather than a fall, in this venous pressure during inspiration. This is termed *Kussmaul's sign* and is seen in constrictive pericardial disease and not in pericardial effusion. It is due to a failure of transmission of negative intrathoracic pressure through the rigid pericardium to the heart.

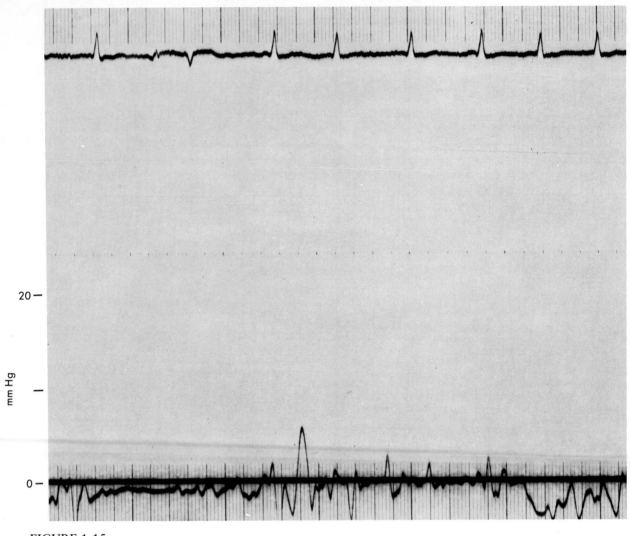

FIGURE 1-15

ANALYSIS

Rhythm: Atrial fibrillation

Pressure(s): (?)

Waveform characteristics and measurements:

1.	;	_____ mm Hg
2.	;	_____ mm Hg
3.	;	_____ mm Hg
4.	;	_____ mm Hg
5.	;	_____ mm Hg
6.	;	_____ mm Hg
7.	;	_____ mm Hg

Suspected abnormality/diagnosis: Loose connection

Comments:

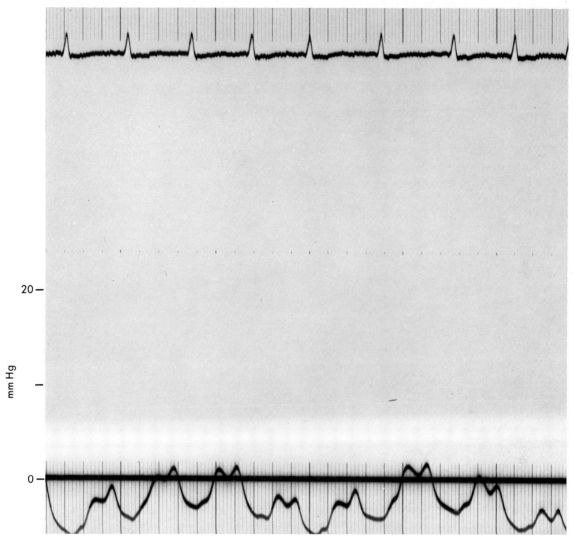

FIGURE 1-16

ANALYSIS

Rhythm: Atrial fibrillation

Pressure(s): (?) Possibly RA

Waveform characteristics and measurements:

1. _____ ; _____ mm Hg
2. _____ ; _____ mm Hg
3. _____ ; _____ mm Hg
4. _____ ; _____ mm Hg
5. _____ ; _____ mm Hg
6. _____ ; _____ mm Hg
7. _____ ; _____ mm Hg

Suspected abnormality/diagnosis: Inaccurate RA pressure due to placement of the transducer air reference level above the level of the patient's right atrium

Comments:

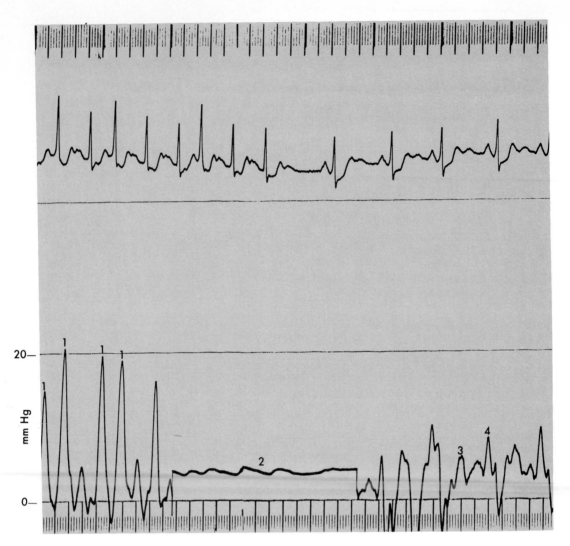

FIGURE 1-17

ANALYSIS

Rhythm: Atrial flutter NSR

Pressure(s): RA

Waveform characteristics and measurements:

1.	Cannon *a* Wave	;	18	mm Hg
2.	Mean	;	4	mm Hg
3.	*a* Wave	;	6	mm Hg
4.	*v* Wave	;	8	mm Hg
5.		;		mm Hg
6.		;		mm Hg
7.		;		mm Hg

Suspected abnormality/diagnosis: Normal right atrial response to atrial flutter

Comments: In the initial portion of this tracing, the patient is in atrial flutter (2:1) with the RA waveform revealing giant or cannon *a* waves whenever the atrium contracts against the closed tricuspid valve. The *a* wave becomes normal when the patient is in sinus rhythm as in the last portion of this tracing.

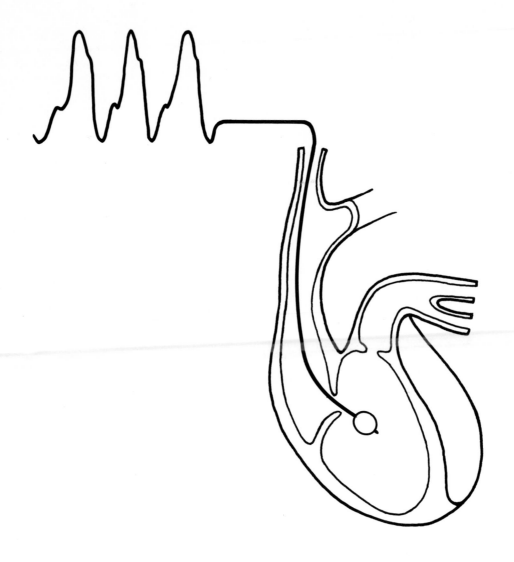

Chapter 2

Right Ventricular Pressures

Physiology and Morphology

The pressure changes in the right ventricle reflect the dynamic, pumping action of that chamber. In general, the phases are systole and diastole; however, these are broken down into seven specific events that constitute ventricular dynamics (Figure 2-1).

Systolic events
1. Isovolumetric contraction
2. Rapid ejection
3. Reduced ejection

Diastolic events
4. Isovlumetric relaxation
5. Early diastole
6. Atrial systole (kick)
7. End-diastole

Isovolumetric contraction refers to the increase in tension or pressure due to ventricular muscle contraction without any change in ventricular volume. ("Iso" means equal; "volumetric" refers to volume.) This is because both the tricuspid and pulmonic valves are closed during this time. The continued rise in ventricular pressure, however, forces the pulmonic valve open, and *rapid ejection* of blood into the pulmonary artery occurs. *Reduced ejection* is characterized by a drop in ventricular pressure, even though some blood is still being pumped into the PA.

Diastole occurs when the ventricular pressure has dropped lower than the PA pressure, causing the pulmonic valve to close. This sharp decline in pressure is due to *isovolumetric relaxation.* The ventricular muscle fibers are relaxing and losing tension while both pulmonic and tricuspid valves are closed, obviating any changes in ventricular volume. When the ventricular diastolic pressure falls below the RA pressure, the tricuspid valve opens, resulting in passive filling of the right ventricle. This period is termed *early diastole* or the rapid filling phase. This is soon followed by atrial systole, which forces an additional volume (anywhere from 10% to 15%) of blood into the ventricle. It is evidenced by an increase in pressure, termed the *atrial kick* or simply the *a* wave.

The period immediately succeeding the *a* wave, just before the systolic pressure rise occurs, is termed *end-diastole*. The pressure during this period reflects the end-diastolic volume, the preload of the right side of the heart. It is the ventricular end-diastolic volume that determines the extent of fiber shortening and the subsequent stroke volume according to the Starling law.

The normal RV systolic pressure in only 20 to 30 mm Hg, about one-sixth the pressure generated by the left ventricle (LV). The RV diastolic pressure typically declines to or near zero while the end-diastolic ranges between 5 to 8 mm Hg.

ECG Correlation

The systolic ejection phase of the RV waveform corresponds to ventricular depolarization, or more generally the QT interval of the ECG. The diastolic period occurs, generally, in the TQ period of the ECG.

Abnormal Findings

Elevation of the RV systolic pressure occurs with pulmonary hypertension (whatever the cause), VSD, or pulmonic stenosis. Normally the RV and PA systolic pressures are essentially equal. In pulmonic stenosis the RV systolic pressure is much greater than the PA systolic pressure due to the resistance to ejection met at the narrowed pulmonic valve.

The RV diastolic pressure is elevated in right ventricular failure, constrictive pericarditis, or cardiac tamponade. Left-sided heart failure of long standing may also be reflected back as an increase in RVedp.

RV pressure is usually not directly monitored at the bedside. However, it is indirectly monitored through evaluation of the PA systolic pressure, which equals RV systolic pressure, and the RA mean pressure, which approximates the RV end-diastolic pressure (if either tricuspid or pulmonic valvular disease is not present). Knowledge of the events producing the RV pressure waveform is useful, since the same physiologic events produce the left ventricular pressure. Accurate identification of RV pressure waveform is essential for safe, accurate hemodynamic monitoring. The presence of an RV pressure waveform on the oscilloscope (Figure 2-5) requires withdrawal of the catheter to the RA or inflation of the balloon for flotation of the catheter out to the PA.

EXAMPLES

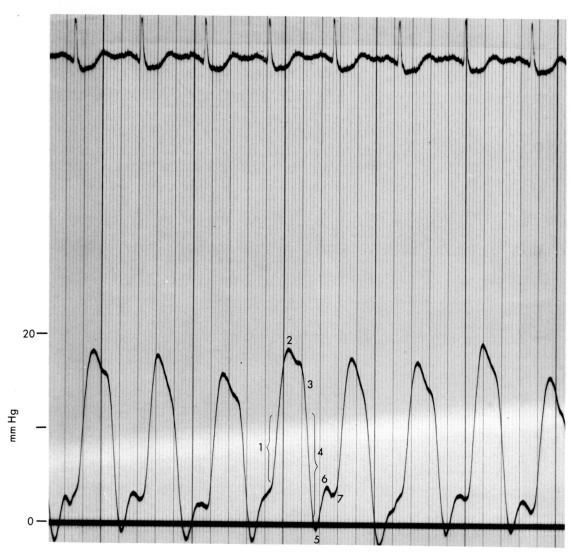

FIGURE 2-1

ANALYSIS

Rhythm: NSR

Pressure(s): RV

Waveform characteristics and measurements:

1.	Isovolumetric contraction	;	_____ mm Hg
2.	Rapid ejection	;	_____ mm Hg
3.	Reduced ejection	;	_____ mm Hg
4.	Isovolumetric relaxation	;	_____ mm Hg
5.	Early diastole	;	_____ mm Hg
6.	Atrial systole	;	_____ mm Hg
7.	End-diastole	;	_____ mm Hg

Suspected abnormality/diagnosis: Normal

Comments: Note the early diastolic pressure falling to baseline and below.

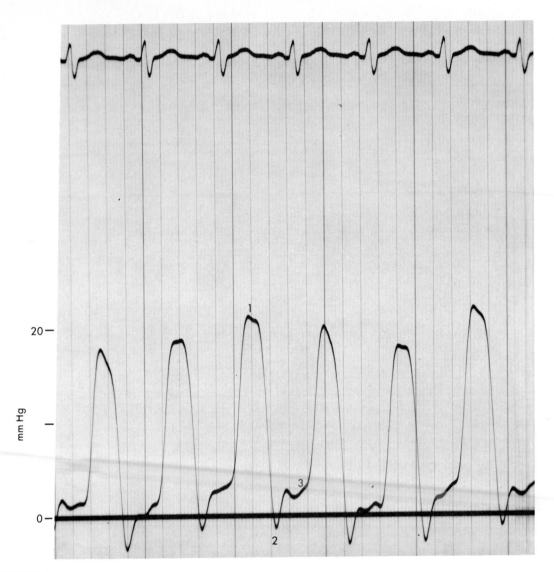

FIGURE 2-2

ANALYSIS

Rhythm: NSR

Pressure(s): RV

Waveform characteristics and measurements:

1.	RV systolic	;	20	mm Hg
2.	RV early diastolic dip	;		mm Hg
3.	RV end-diastolic	;	2	mm Hg
4.		;		mm Hg
5.		;		mm Hg
6.		;		mm Hg
7.		;		mm Hg

Suspected abnormality/diagnosis: Normal

Comments:

26

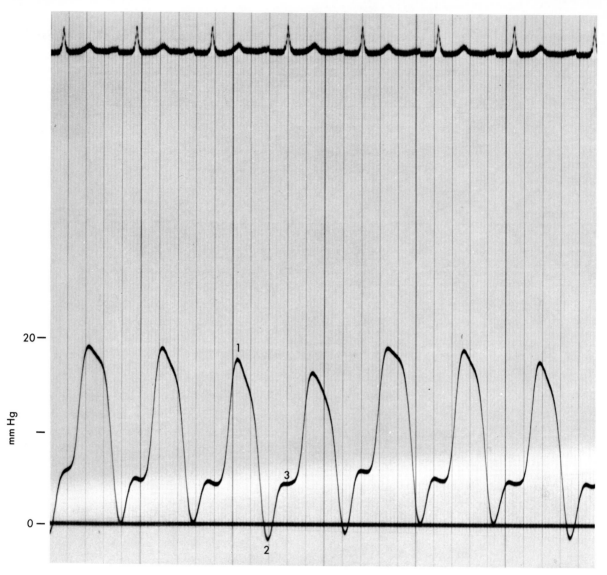

FIGURE 2-3

ANALYSIS

Rhythm: NSR

Pressure(s): RV

Waveform characteristics and measurements:

1.	RV systolic	;	18	mm Hg
2.	RV diastolic dip	;	0	mm Hg
3.	RV end-diastolic	;	5	mm Hg
4.		;		mm Hg
5.		;		mm Hg
6.		;		mm Hg
7.		;		mm Hg

Suspected abnormality/diagnosis: Normal

Comments:

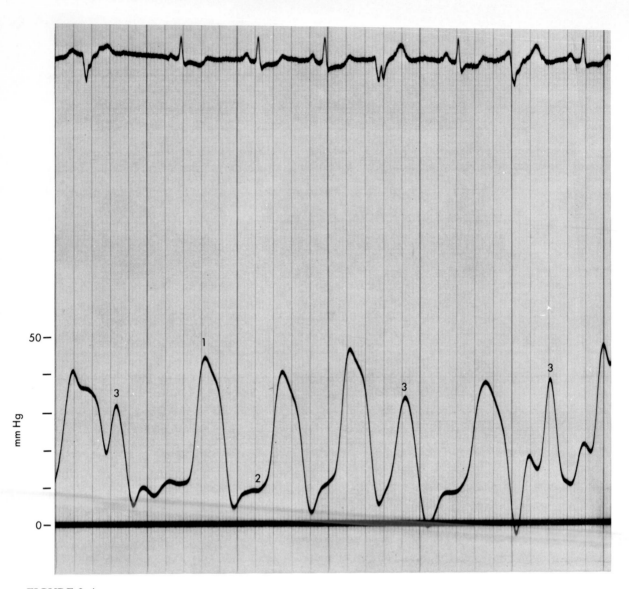

FIGURE 2-4

ANALYSIS

Rhythm: NSR with PVCs

Pressure(s): RV

Waveform characteristics and measurements:

1.	RV systolic	; 40	mm Hg
2.	RV end-diastolic	; 11	mm Hg
3.	PVC	;	mm Hg
4.		;	mm Hg
5.		;	mm Hg
6.		;	mm Hg
7.		;	mm Hg

Suspected abnormality/diagnosis: Right-sided heart failure

Comments: Note the reduced ejection following the PVCs. The elevated end-diastolic pressure of 11 mm Hg indicates RV failure; the elevated systolic pressure of 40 mm Hg suggests that the failure may be due to an increase in resistance to ejection either from pulmonary disease, mitral valve disease, or left-sided heart failure.

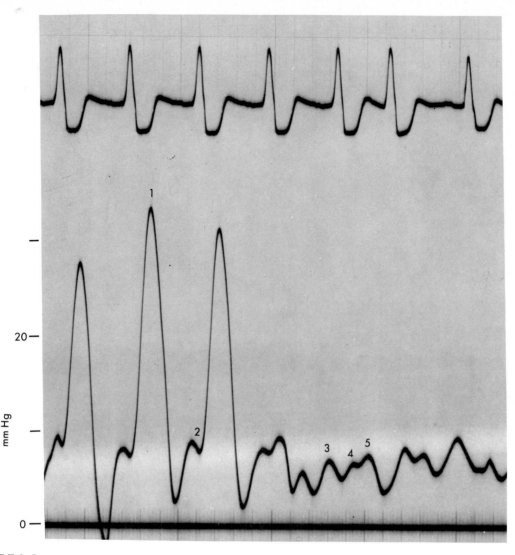

FIGURE 2-5

ANALYSIS

Rhythm: NSR with APC

Pressure(s): RV to RA

Waveform characteristics and measurements:

1.	RV systolic	;	30	mm Hg
2.	RV end-diastolic	;	8	mm Hg
3.	RA *a* wave	;	8	mm Hg
4.	RA *c* wave	;		mm Hg
5.	RA *v* wave	;	8	mm Hg
6.	RA mean	;	6	mm Hg
7.		;		mm Hg

Suspected abnormality/diagnosis: Mild RV failure

Comments: Note the similarity between the RV end-diastolic pressure *(2)* and the RA *a* wave *(3)*.

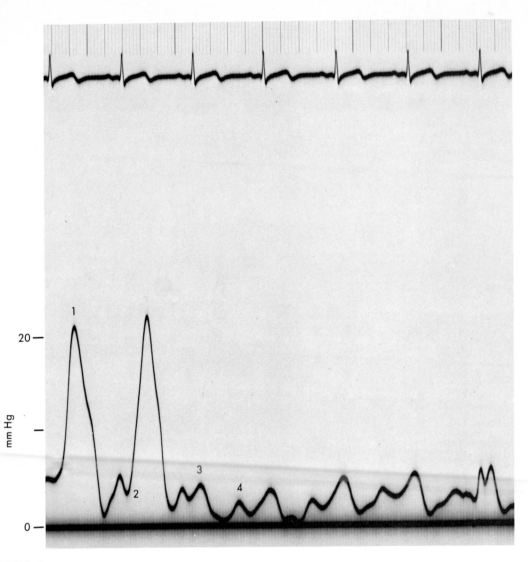

FIGURE 2-6

ANALYSIS

Rhythm: NSR

Pressure(s): RV to RA

Waveform characteristics and measurements:

1.	RV systolic	;	22	mm Hg
2.	RV end-diastolic	;	3	mm Hg
3.	RA *a* wave	;	3	mm Hg
4.	RA *v* wave	;	2	mm Hg
5.	RA mean	;	3	mm Hg
6.		;		mm Hg
7.		;		mm Hg

Suspected abnormality/diagnosis: Normal RV and RA pressures.

Comments:

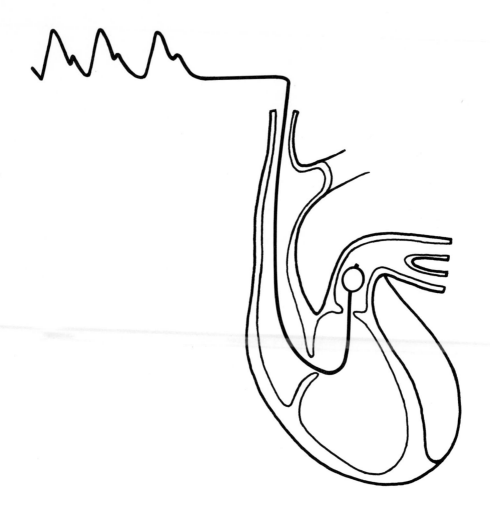

Chapter 3

Pulmonary Artery Pressures

Physiology and Morphology

The pulmonary artery (PA) pressure is divided into two phases: systole and diastole. Systole begins with the opening of the pulmonic valve, resulting in rapid ejection of blood into the pulmonary artery. On the PA pressure tracing this is seen as a sharp rise in pressure, followed by a decline in pressure as the volume decreases (Figure 3-1). When the RV pressure falls below the level of the PA pressure, the pulmonic valve snaps shut. This sudden closure of the valve leaflets produces a small notch on the downslope of the PA pressure and is termed the *dicrotic notch*. The systolic value referred to is the peak systolic pressure reached. Normal PA systolic pressure is 20 to 30 mm Hg (the same as the RV systolic pressure).

Diastole follows closure of the pulmonic valve. During this time, runoff to the pulmonary system occurs without any further blood flow from the right ventricle until the next systolic ejection. The PA diastolic value referred to is the end-diastolic pressure just prior to the next systole. This value corresponds closely to the LV end-diastolic pressure (LVedp) in the absence of pulmonary disease or mitral valve disease. Normal PA end-diastolic pressure is 8 to 12 mm Hg.

ECG Correlation

The systolic phase of the PA pressure should correspond closely to ventricular depolarization. However, catheter length and the amount of tubing used can delay this somewhat. Generally, it occurs in the QT interval of the ECG. The dicrotic notch occurs after the T wave of the ECG.

In atrial fibrillation the value of the PA pressure varies greatly (Figure 3-8), depending on the RR intervals and length of time for ventricular filling. The shorter the RR interval, the shorter the ventricular filling time, the less stroke volume ejected, and the less pressure rise in the PA. The contour of the PA pressure tracing remains normal, however.

Abnormal Findings

Certain pathologic conditions alter the PA pressure. Elevation of the PA pressure occurs with increased pulmonary vascular resistance (PVR), increased pulmonary venous pressure, and increased pulmonary blood flow. Pulmonary disease, essential pulmonary hypertension, and hypoxia elevate the PA pressure due to an increase in pulmonary vascular resistance. Mitral valve disease and LV failure increase pulmonary venous pressure which in turn increases the PA pressure. Intracardiac left-to-right shunts, either atrial or ventricular, increase pulmonary blood flow and PA pressure.

In general, the PAedp correlates closely with the PAW pressure. This allows us to more safely monitor the PAedp as a reflection of LVedp and avoid obtaining repeated PAW pressures with its inherent risks of damage to the pulmonary vasculature, including hemorrhage, ischemia, and pulmonary infarction. There are some situations, however, in which there is a wide discrepancy between the PAedp and PAW pressures. As mentioned previously, pulmonary disease elevates pulmonary artery pressure but usually does not affect the PAW pressure, which is a reflection of LA pressure, that is distal to the level of increased resistance. Pulmonary embolus also increases resistance and therefore increases PA pressure without affecting the PAW pressure. Very rapid heart rates elevate the PA diastolic pressure by abbreviating the duration of the diastolic period. In all these situations it may be necessary to use the PAW pressure to monitor LVedp.

Occasionally, the presence of giant v waves in the PAW pressure wave may be transmitted back onto the PA pressure distorting the contour of the PA waveform, giving it an almost bifid appearance. At times, the transmitted v wave may be even higher than the PA systolic pressure producing a very unusual PA waveform. Careful assessment of the timing of the v wave with the patient's ECG and the PAW pressure are necessary to discern these phenomena.

In addition to pathologic abnormalities, mechanical abnormalities frequently alter the PA pressure both in contour and value. "Fling" or "whip" in the PA pressure tracing (Figure 3-5), consisting of exaggerated oscillations, can occur with excessive catheter coiling in either the right atrium or right ventricle or when the catheter tip is located near the pulmonic valve, where blood flow is turbulent. Patients with pulmonary hypertension and dilated pulmonary arteries frequently exhibit fling in the PA pressure tracing. In these situations accurate measurement of the PA pressure is difficult, and manipulation and repositioning of the catheter are necessary.

Damping of the PA pressure, due to a variety of causes, changes both the contour and the value of the PA waveform in a characteristic manner (Figure 3-3). The entire waveform loses any sharp definition and becomes rather rounded out in appearance. Frequently the upstroke of the systolic pressure is slow and the dicrotic notch is absent or poorly defined. The value of the PA pressure is decreased considerably and as such is an inaccurate pressure. Most often fibrin at the tip of the catheter is the culprit when pressures become damped. Careful aspiration followed by gentle flushing usually corrects this problem, but occasionally catheter replacement is necessary. Placement of the tip of the catheter against the wall of the vessel also produces damped pressures and requires repositioning of the catheter. The presence of an air bubble(s) anywhere within the system also dampens the pressure waveform. Kinks in either the catheter itself or the extension tubing produce a dampened, lowered pressure waveform.

EXAMPLES

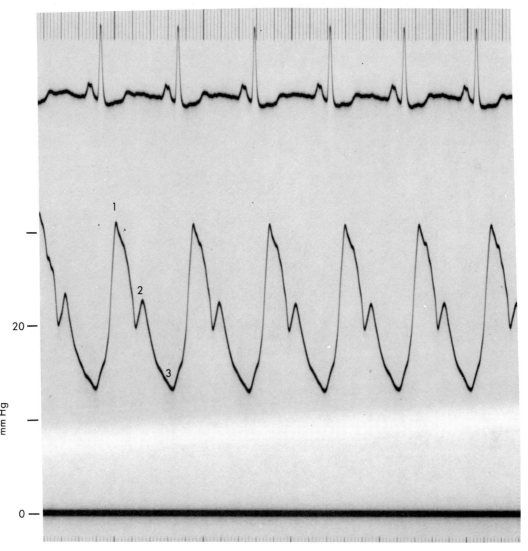

FIGURE 3-1

ANALYSIS

Rhythm: NSR

Pressure(s): PA

Waveform characteristics and measurements:

1.	PA systolic	; 30	mm Hg
2.	Dicrotic notch	;	mm Hg
3.	PA end-diastolic	; 13	mm Hg
4.		;	mm Hg
5.		;	mm Hg
6.		;	mm Hg
7.		;	mm Hg

Suspected abnormality/diagnosis: Normal

Comments:

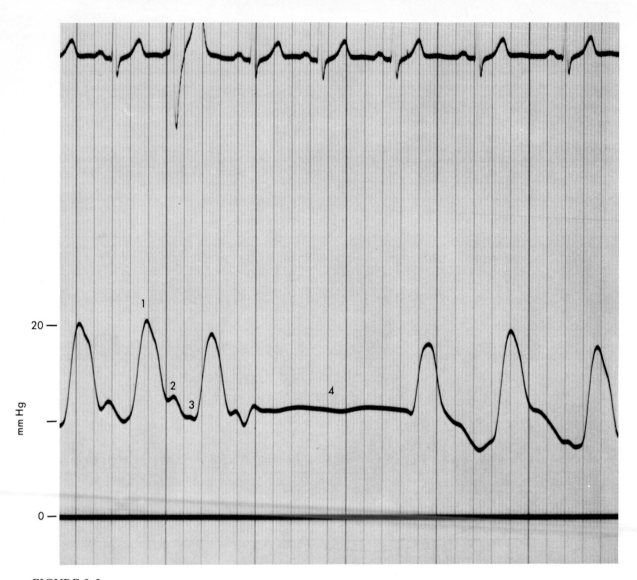

FIGURE 3-2

ANALYSIS

Rhythm: NSR with PVC

Pressure(s): PA

Waveform characteristics and measurements:

1.	PA systolic	;	20	mm Hg
2.	Dicrotic notch	;		mm Hg
3.	PA end-diastolic	;	9	mm Hg
4.	Electrical mean	;	12	mm Hg
5.		;		mm Hg
6.		;		mm Hg
7.		;		mm Hg

Suspected abnormality/diagnosis: Normal

Comments: Because diastole comprises approximately two thirds of the cardiac cycle, the average or mean of the PA pressure is much closer to the diastolic value than the systolic value.

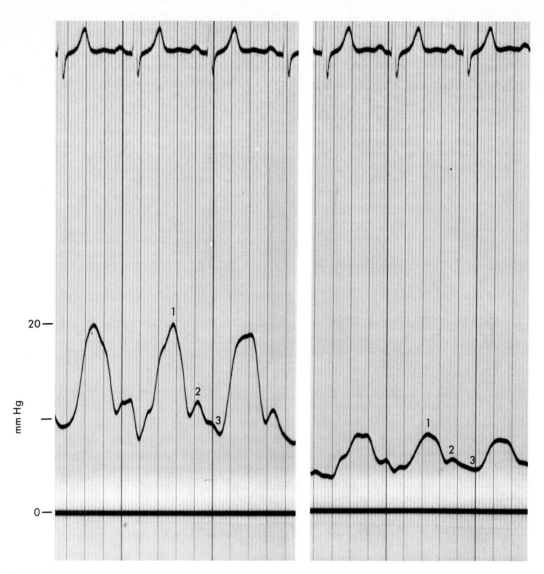

FIGURE 3-3

ANALYSIS

Rhythm: NSR

Pressure(s): PA

Waveform characteristics and measurements:

1.	PA systolic	; 20 (8)	mm Hg
2.	Dicrotic notch	;	mm Hg
3.	PA end-diastolic	; 9 (4)	mm Hg
4.		;	mm Hg
5.		;	mm Hg
6.		;	mm Hg
7.		;	mm Hg

Suspected abnormality/diagnosis: Normal and damped

Comments: Note the damping effect in the latter three pressure waveforms due to a clot at the tip of the catheter or an air bubble within the system. Note the similar contour of the pressure tracings, with a marked decrease in value.

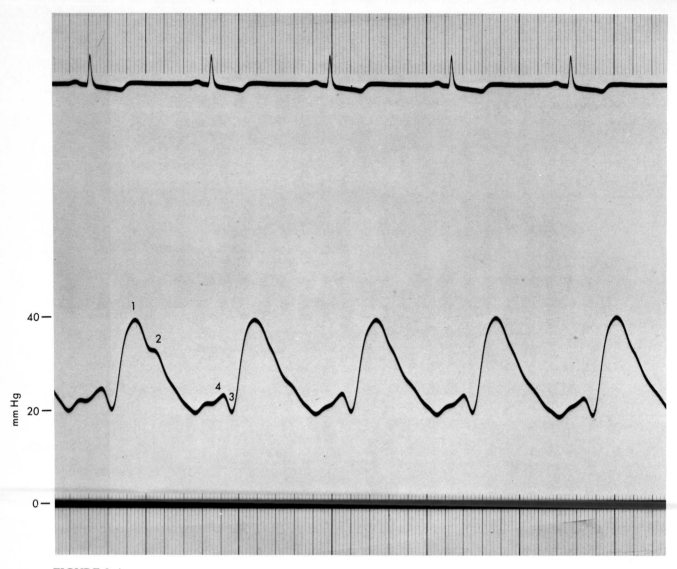

FIGURE 3-4

ANALYSIS

Rhythm: NSR

Pressure(s): PA

Waveform characteristics and measurements:

1.	PA systolic	; 40	mm Hg
2.	Dicrotic notch	;	mm Hg
3.	*a* Wave reflected back from LA	;	mm Hg
4.	PA end-diastolic	; 20	mm Hg
5.		;	mm Hg
6.		;	mm Hg
7.		;	mm Hg

Suspected abnormality/diagnosis: Mild CHF

Comments: This PA pressure waveform is somewhat damped with a rounded-out appearance and poorly defined dicrotic notch. It is possible, at times, to see retrograde transmission of the LA *a* wave.

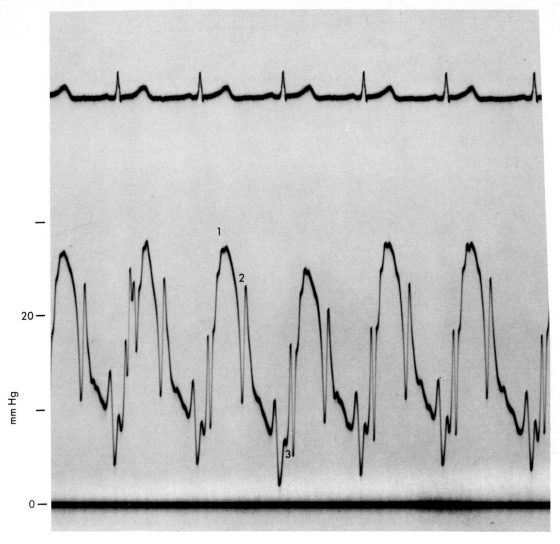

FIGURE 3-5

ANALYSIS

Rhythm: NSR

Pressure(s): PA

Waveform characteristics and measurements:

1.	PA systolic	;	26	mm Hg
2.	Dicrotic notch	;		mm Hg
3.	PA end-diastolic	;	(?) 9	mm Hg
4.		;		mm Hg
5.		;		mm Hg
6.		;		mm Hg
7.		;		mm Hg

Suspected abnormality/diagnosis: Normal

Comments: This PA pressure is of normal value, however, the contour is abnormal due to catheter "fling," making accurate identification of PA end-diastolic pressure difficult. The catheter tip is, likely, located near the pulmonic valve and rests in an area of increased turbulence.

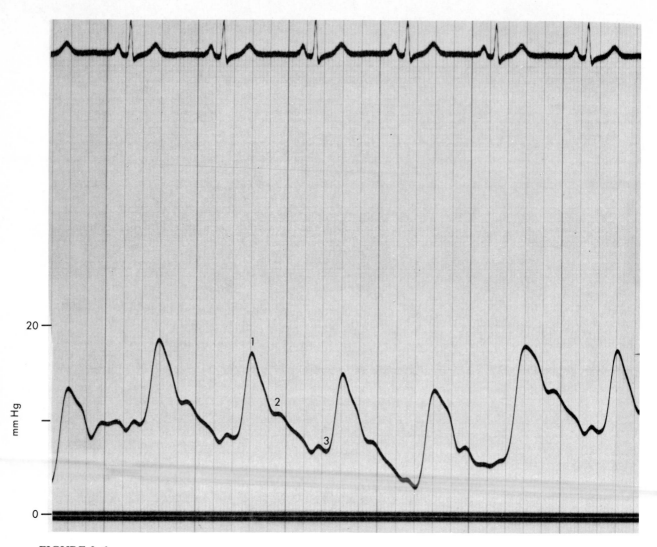

FIGURE 3-6

ANALYSIS

Rhythm: NSR

Pressure(s): PA

Waveform characteristics and measurements:

1.	Systolic	;	15	mm Hg
2.	Dicrotic notch	;		mm Hg
3.	End-diastolic	;	7	mm Hg
4.		;		mm Hg
5.		;		mm Hg
6.		;		mm Hg
7.		;		mm Hg

Suspected abnormality/diagnosis: Normal PA pressure

Comments:

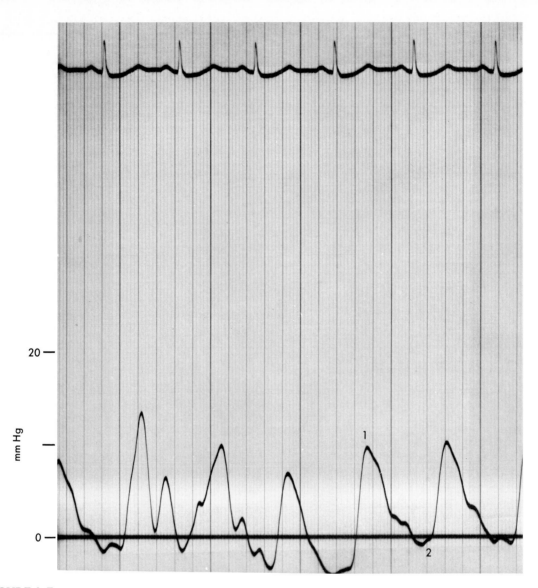

FIGURE 3-7
================

ANALYSIS

Rhythm: NSR

Pressure(s): PA

Waveform characteristics and measurements:

1.	PA systolic	;	10	mm Hg
2.	PA diastolic	;	0	mm Hg
3.		;		mm Hg
4.		;		mm Hg
5.		;		mm Hg
6.		;		mm Hg
7.		;		mm Hg

Suspected abnormality/diagnosis: Artifactual pressure

Comments: This artifactually low pressure is due to incorrect placement of the transducer air-reference level above the level of the right atrium. Because the diastolic pressure falls to or even below the baseline (zero), this PA pressure tracing could be confused with an RV pressure tracing. However, closer scrutiny reveals a normal PA contour with systole, dicrotic notch, and runoff in diastole.

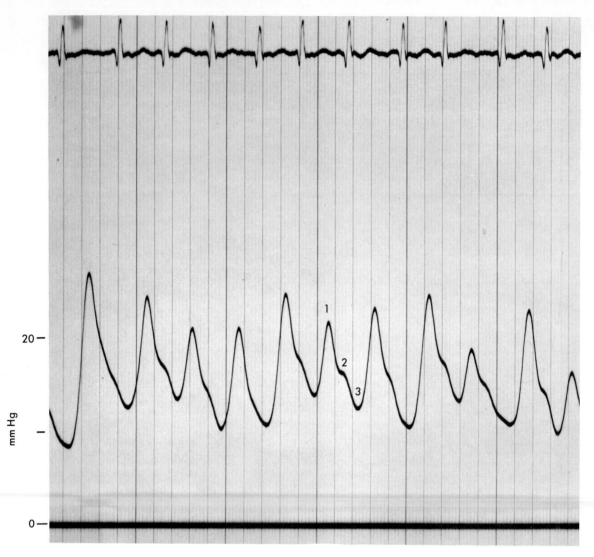

FIGURE 3-8

ANALYSIS

Rhythm: Rapid atrial fibrillation

Pressure(s): PA

Waveform characteristics and measurements:

1.	PA systolic	;	19-24	mm Hg
2.	Dicrotic notch	;		mm Hg
3.	PA end-diastolic	;	9-14	mm Hg
4.		;		mm Hg
5.		;		mm Hg
6.		;		mm Hg
7.		;		mm Hg

Suspected abnormality/diagnosis: Normal

Comments: Note varying PA systolic pressure secondary to varying RR intervals and length of time for diastolic filling to occur.

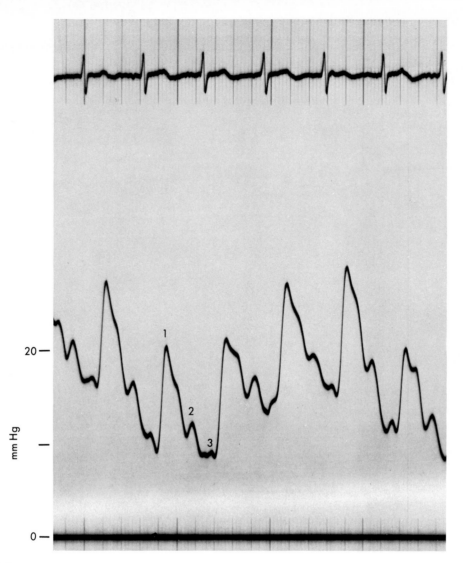

FIGURE 3-9

ANALYSIS

Rhythm: Regular supraventricular tachycardia

Pressure(s): PA

Waveform characteristics and measurements:

1.	PA systolic	; 25	mm Hg
2.	Dicrotic notch	;	mm Hg
3.	PA end-diastolic	; 12	mm Hg
4.		;	mm Hg
5.		;	mm Hg
6.		;	mm Hg
7.		;	mm Hg

Suspected abnormality/diagnosis: Normal

Comments: Note the exaggerated, but normal, respiratory variation in this PA pressure tracing, with the end-diastolic value ranging from a low of 9 mm Hg to a high of 15 mm Hg. A more accurate reading can be obtained by measuring the PA pressure at the very end of expiration.

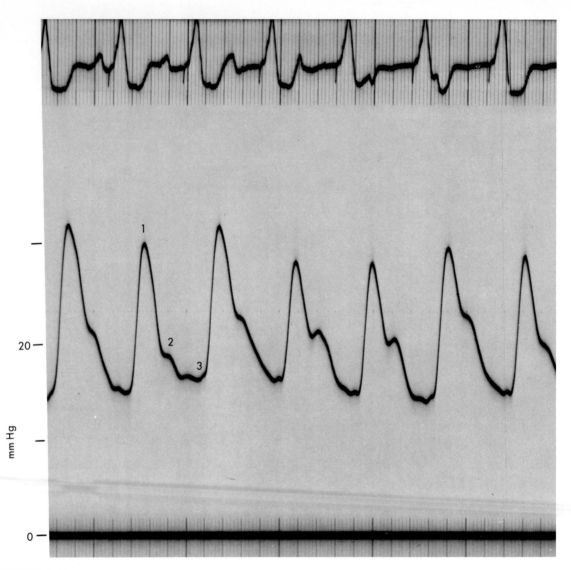

FIGURE 3-10

ANALYSIS

Rhythm: Paced (Note pacemaker spikes and P waves throughout ECG).

Pressure(s): PA

Waveform characteristics and measurements:

1.	PA systolic	;	31	mm Hg
2.	Dicrotic notch	;		mm Hg
3.	PA end-diastolic	;	16	mm Hg
4.		;		mm Hg
5.		;		mm Hg
6.		;		mm Hg
7.		;		mm Hg

Suspected abnormality/diagnosis: Mild pulmonary hypertension

Comments:

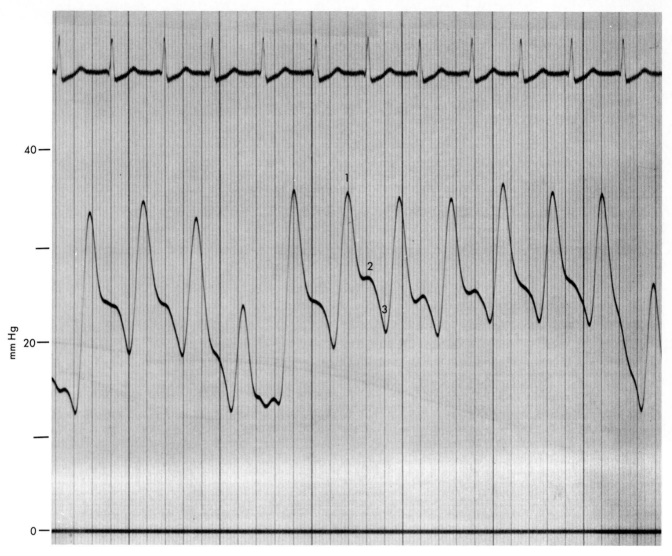

FIGURE 3-11

ANALYSIS

Rhythm: Sinus tachycardia

Pressure(s): PA

Waveform characteristics and measurements:

1.	PA systolic	;	35	mm Hg
2.	Dicrotic notch	;		mm Hg
3.	PA end-diastolic	;	20	mm Hg
4.		;		mm Hg
5.		;		mm Hg
6.		;		mm Hg
7.		;		mm Hg

Suspected abnormality/diagnosis: Pulmonary hypertension secondary to pulmonary disease

Comments: The mildly elevated PA pressure of 35/20 is due to increased PVR as a result of pulmonary disease. This pressure does not reflect left-sided heart pressures. Therefore the PAW pressure, instead of the PAedp, should be monitored to reflect LVedp. Note the marked drop in PA pressure during brief inspiration.

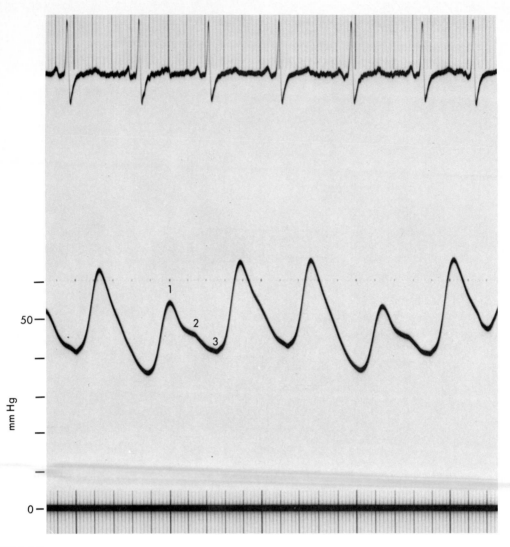

FIGURE 3-12

ANALYSIS

Rhythm: NSR

Pressure(s): PA

Waveform characteristics and measurements:

1.	PA systolic	;	60	mm Hg
2.	Dicrotic notch	;		mm Hg
3.	PA end-diastolic	;	40	mm Hg
4.		;		mm Hg
5.		;		mm Hg
6.		;		mm Hg
7.		;		mm Hg

Suspected abnormality/diagnosis: Pulmonary hypertension

Comments: This PA waveform appears damped, a frequent finding in patients with high PVR. Note pressure changes due to respiratory variation.

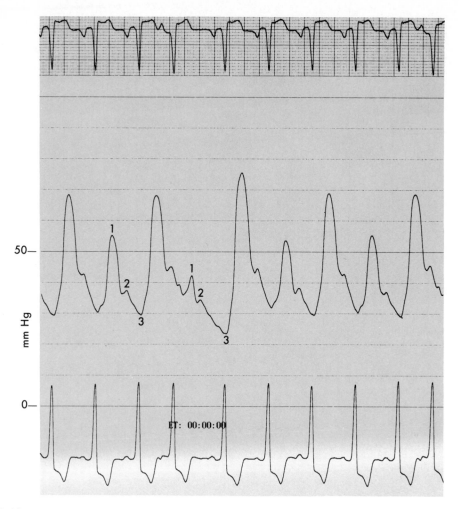

FIGURE 3-13

ANALYSIS

Rhythm: Sinus tachycardia

Pressure(s): PA

Waveform characteristics and measurements:

1.	Systolic	;	51-70	mm Hg
2.	Dicrotic notch	;		mm Hg
3.	Diastolic	;	30	mm Hg
4.		;		mm Hg
5.		;		mm Hg
6.		;		mm Hg
7.		;		mm Hg

Suspected abnormality/diagnosis: Pulmonary hypertension secondary to CHF

Comments: Note the regular, alternating reduction in the PA systolic pressure. This is due to pulsus alternans with regular changes in the stroke volume of the right heart with every other beat. This usually is associated with severe ventricular failure.

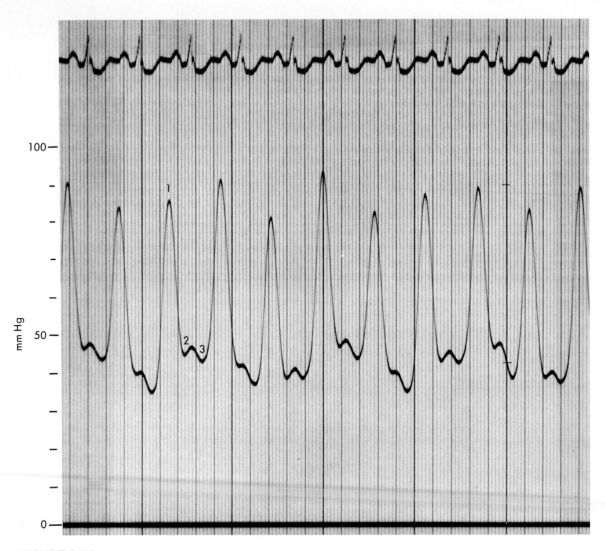

FIGURE 3-14

ANALYSIS

Rhythm: Sinus tachycardia

Pressure(s): PA

Waveform characteristics and measurements:

1.	PA systolic	; 87	mm Hg
2.	Dicrotic notch	;	mm Hg
3.	PA end-diastolic	; 40	mm Hg
4.		;	mm Hg
5.		;	mm Hg
6.		;	mm Hg
7.		;	mm Hg

Suspected abnormality/diagnosis: Pulmonary hypertension secondary to severe mitral stenosis and mitral regurgitation

Comments: Note the abbreviated diastolic phase due to the tachycardia. This shortened diastolic period causes the pressure to remain high at end-diastole and not correspond to the PAW mean or LV end-diastolic pressures.

48

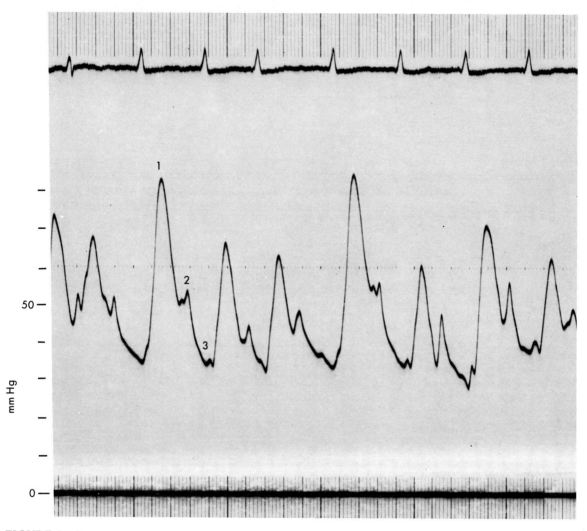

FIGURE 3-15

ANALYSIS

Rhythm: Atrial fibrillation

Pressure(s): PA

Waveform characteristics and measurements:

1.	PA systolic	;	72	mm Hg
2.	Dicrotic notch	;		mm Hg
3.	PA end-diastolic	;	32	mm Hg
4.		;		mm Hg
5.		;		mm Hg
6.		;		mm Hg
7.		;		mm Hg

Suspected abnormality/diagnosis: Severe pulmonary hypertension secondary to mitral regurgitation and CHF

Comments: Note the broadened dicrotic notch which is distorted as a result of the retrograde reflection of the LA or PAW *v* wave of 45 to 55 mm Hg secondary to severe mitral regurgitation.

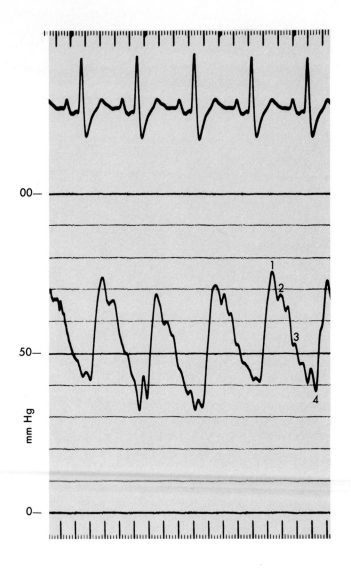

FIGURE 3-16

ANALYSIS

Rhythm: NSR

Pressure(s): PA

Waveform characteristics and measurements:

1.	Systolic	;	70	mm Hg
2.	Retrograde *v* wave	;		mm Hg
3.	Dicrotic notch	;		mm Hg
4.	End-diastolic	;	40	mm Hg
5.		;		mm Hg
6.		;		mm Hg
7.		;		mm Hg

Suspected abnormality/diagnosis: Pulmonary hypertension secondary to mitral regurgitation

Comments: The appearance of this elevated PA waveform is altered by the retrograde reflection of the LA *v* wave due to severe mitral regurgitation. In timing, this event follows the T wave of the ECG.

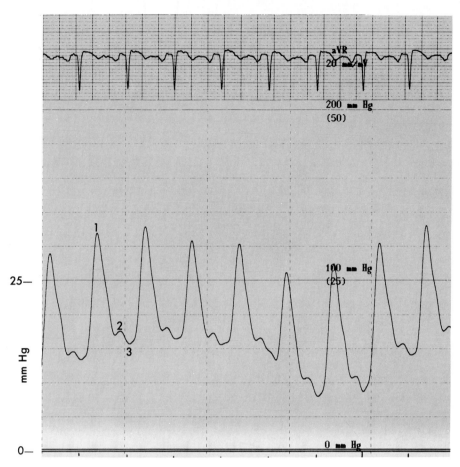

FIGURE 3-17

ANALYSIS

Rhythm: Sinus tachycardia

Pressure(s): PA

Waveform characteristics and measurements:

1.	Systolic	;	30	mm Hg
2.	Dicrotic notch	;		mm Hg
3.	Diastolic	;	14	mm Hg
4.		;		mm Hg
5.		;		mm Hg
6.		;		mm Hg
7.		;		mm Hg

Suspected abnormality/diagnosis: Mild pulmonary hypertension

Comments: This PA pressure is mildly elevated with a very abbreviated diastolic period due to the rapid heart rate.

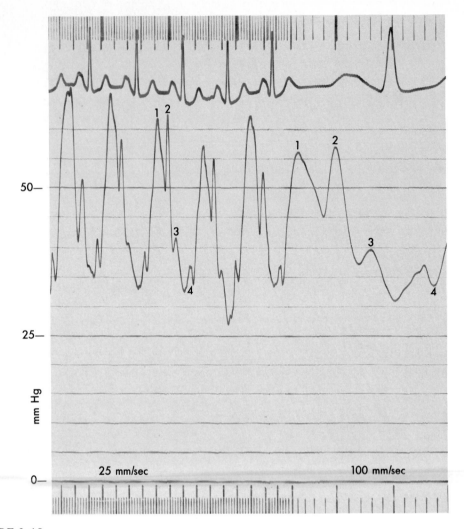

FIGURE 3-18

ANALYSIS

Rhythm: NSR

Pressure(s): PA

Waveform characteristics and measurements:

1.	Systolic	;	70	mm Hg
2.	Retrograde v wave	;	65	mm Hg
3.	Dicrotic notch	;		mm Hg
4.	Diastolic	;	38	mm Hg
5.		;		mm Hg
6.		;		mm Hg
7.		;		mm Hg

Suspected abnormality/diagnosis: Pulmonary hypertension secondary to mitral regurgitation

Comments: The first notch following the systolic peak of this PA waveform represents the LA v wave reflected onto the PA waveform. Note its appropriate timing following the T wave of the ECG. This is more easily discerned when the paper speed is increased to 100 mm/sec as in the latter portion of this tracing.

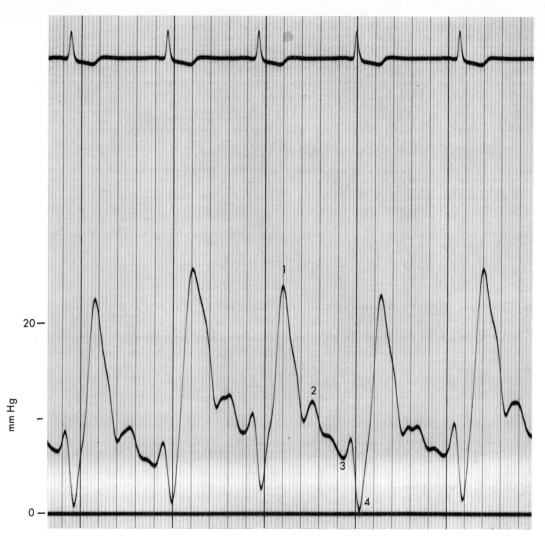

FIGURE 3-19

ANALYSIS

Rhythm: Atrial fibrillation

Pressure(s): PA/RV

Waveform characteristics and measurements:

1.	PA systolic	;	24	mm Hg
2.	Dicrotic notch	;		mm Hg
3.	PA end-diastolic	;	9	mm Hg
4.	RV diastolic	;	1	mm Hg
5.		;		mm Hg
6.		;		mm Hg
7.		;		mm Hg

Suspected abnormality/diagnosis: Normal

Comments: The contour of this pressure waveform has the appearance of a mixed PA/RV pressure with the diastolic pressure coming down to baseline. This is due to location of the catheter tip right at the pulmonic valve, which results in forward movement of the catheter into the PA during systole and backward movement of the catheter into the RV during diastole. Inflation of the balloon of the catheter should allow the catheter to float out to the PA.

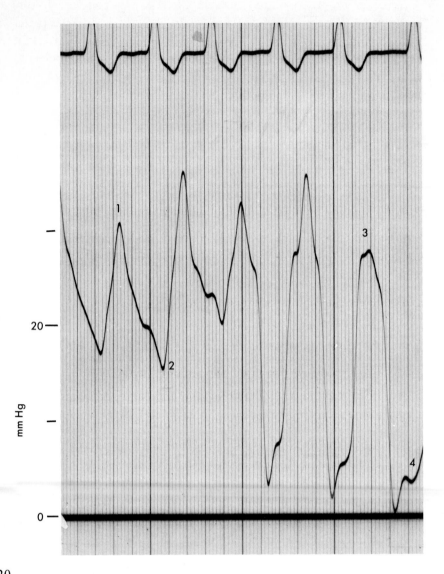

FIGURE 3-20

ANALYSIS

Rhythm: Atrial fibrillation

Pressure(s): PA to RV

Waveform characteristics and measurements:

1.	PA systolic	;	32	mm Hg
2.	PA end-diastolic	;	18	mm Hg
3.	RV systolic	;	30	mm Hg
4.	RV end-diastolic	;	6	mm Hg
5.		;		mm Hg
6.		;		mm Hg
7.		;		mm Hg

Suspected abnormality/diagnosis: Normal

Comments: The catheter has slipped from the PA back into the RV. Inflation of the balloon should carry the tip of the catheter back into the PA. If this does not occur, the catheter must be withdrawn out of the RV. Note the normal respiratory variation in both pressures.

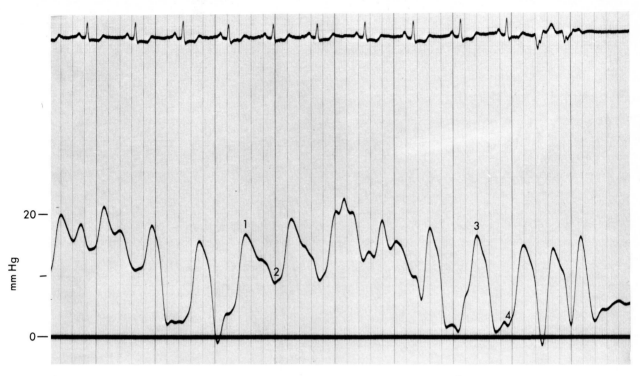

FIGURE 3-21

ANALYSIS

Rhythm: NSR with PVCs

Pressure(s): PA and RV

Waveform characteristics and measurements:

1.	PA systolic	;	19	mm Hg
2.	PA end-diastolic	;	10	mm Hg
3.	RV systolic	;	17	mm Hg
4.	RV end-diastolic	;	2	mm Hg
5.		;		mm Hg
6.		;		mm Hg
7.		;		mm Hg

Suspected abnormality/diagnosis: Normal

Comments: The tip of the catheter is located at the pulmonic valve, moving back and forth across the valve and producing PA and RV pressure waveforms. It is not in a safe location for monitoring purposes (note the occurrence of PVCs). It would also be impossible to obtain a PAW pressure waveform with the catheter tip in this location. Usually inflation of the balloon will carry the catheter tip distally out to the PA. Unfortunately it is usually not carried distally enough to obtain a PAW pressure, but safe monitoring of the PA pressure can be continued.

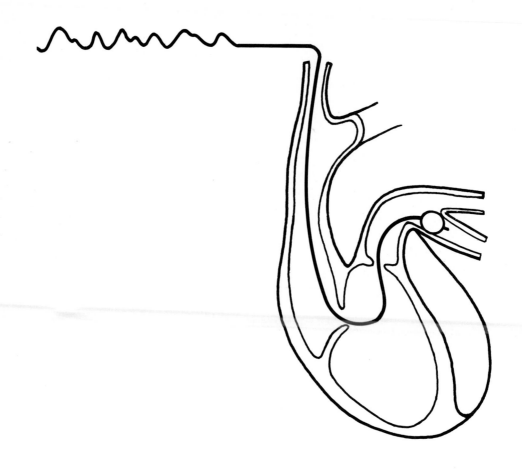

Chapter 4

Pulmonary Artery Wedge Pressures

Physiology and Morphology

When proper position in a small branch of the PA is achieved, inflation of the balloon of the pulmonary artery catheter actually occludes flow in that segment of the pulmonary artery. The pressure obtained with balloon inflation is termed the pulmonary artery occluded or *pulmonary artery wedge (PAW)* pressure. This pressure reflects left atrial (LA) pressure and has similar contour and characteristics as the right atrial pressure (*a, c,* and *v* waves with *x* and *y* descents) since the pressure is produced by the same physiolgoic events (Figure 4-1). The *a* wave of the PAW pressure is produced by LA systole and is followed by the *x* descent, reflecting left atrial relaxation following systole. The *c* wave that is produced by closure of the mitral valve frequently gets lost in retrograde transmission and often is not observed in the PAW pressure waveform, although it can be seen at times. The *v* wave is produced by filling of the LA and bulging of the mitral valve during ventricular systole. The decline succeeding the *v* wave is the *y* descent, which represents opening of the mitral valve with a decrease in LA pressure and volume during passive emptying into the LV.

Although the contour of the PAW pressure is the same as the RA pressure, the value of the PAW pressure is normally higher. As with the RA pressure, we generally record the mean of the PAW pressure, since the *a* and *v* waves are normally of approximately the same value. The normal resting PAW mean pressure is 4 to 12 mm Hg. If, however, either the *a* or the *v* wave is particularly dominant or elevated, it is not accurate to average the pressure rises. In those instances the value of both the *a* wave and the *v* wave should be noted.

ECG Correlation

Timing of the electrical and mechanical events is the same as with the RA pressure, that is, the *a* wave follows the P wave of the ECG, and the *v* wave follows the T wave of the ECG. However, a greater time delay between electrical and mechanical events is frequently noted with the PAW pressure as it is a measurement of pressures retrogradely transmitted from the LA through the pulmonary venous blood to the catheter tip. Thus, the PAW *a* wave usually can be seen approximately 200 to 240 msecs after the electrocardiographic P wave. The *v* wave occurs well after the T wave of the ECG.

The effects of arrhythmias on the PAW pressure are the same as those discussed with the RA pressure. In atrial fibrillation there are no *a* waves in the PAW pressure waveform, and only a *v* wave follows each T wave. Junctional rhythm or AV dissociation can produce giant or cannon *a* waves in the PAW waveform.

The normal respiratory response can be seen in the PAW pressures with a decline during spontaneous inhalation and a rise during exhalation. The opposite effect occurs with mechanical ventilation. Regardless of the mode of ventilation, all hemodynamic pressures should be measured at end-expiration.

Abnormal Findings

Elevated PAW pressures occur in the following conditions:
1. LV failure
2. Mitral stenosis and/or regurgitation
3. Cardiac tamponade
4. Constrictive pericarditis
5. Volume overload

The *a* wave of the PAW pressure is exaggerated and elevated in any condition that increases the resistance to LV filling. Elevation of the PAW *a* wave with LV failure reflects the increased filling pressure required with elevated LV diastolic pressures (Figure 4-11). In pure mitral stenosis the PAW *a* wave is also dominant and elevated due to the resistance met at the narrowed mitral orifice. It represents the increased force of contraction required to eject blood through the stenotic valve. The *y* descent of the PAW pressure is usually prolonged in mitral stenosis, indicating increased resistance to passive filling of the LV.

The *v* wave of the PAW pressure is exaggerated and elevated with mitral insufficiency due to regurgitation of blood back into the LA during ventricular systole (Figure 4-17). Mitral regurgitation can occur in varying degrees of severity and from a variety of causes. A mildly elevated and dominant *v* wave is commonly seen with LV failure and dilatation. Rheumatic fever or bacterial endocarditis can cause destruction of the valve leaflets and produce chronic mitral regurgitation with mildly or moderately elevated *v* waves. Acute mitral regurgitation, with giant *v* waves, can occur with ruptured papillary muscle following myocardial infarction (Figure 4-20). On a lesser scale, ischemia of the papillary muscle can occur resulting in mild to moderate mitral regurgitation and elevation of the *v* wave.

Occasionally, very large *v* waves are reflected back onto the PA pressure (see discussion page 52). Close inspection of the timing of the PAW waveform in relation to the ECG (best done at fast paper speed) usually reveals the *v* wave following the T wave, whereas the upstroke of the PA systolic pressure usually occurs earlier, and corresponds to the QRS of the ECG.

When giant *v* waves are present in the PAW waveform, the mean PAW pressure may be artifactually elevated and may, indeed, be somewhat higher than the *a* wave of the PAW. In these instances, it is more accurate to record the PAW *a* wave as a reflection of the filling pressure of the LV.

In *cardiac tamponade, constrictive pericardial disease,* and *hypervolemia* the PAW *a* and *v* waves are equally elevated. However, in cardiac tamponade the *x* descent is prominent and the *y* descent attenuated or even absent, whereas in constrictive pericarditis either the *y* descent is prominent or the *x* and *y* descents are equal, giving an **M** pattern to the PAW pressure waveform.

Hypovolemia produces a low PAW pressure. In the normal heart, PAW pressures less than 4 or 5 mm Hg indicate hypovolemia, whereas in the compromised heart, hypovolemia may be present with higher PAW pressures.

Mechanical abnormalities of the PAW pressure produce changes in both the value and the contour of the PAW pressure waveform. *Overwedging,* which is caused by overinflation or eccentric inflation of the balloon of the catheter or an exceedingly distal location of the catheter tip, may produce an artifactually elevated, damped, and inaccurate PAW pressure (Figure 4-8). In addition, there is usually a linear increase in the pressure waveform. (It resembles a line at an approximately 10- to 20-degree angle). Slow, careful, and accurate balloon inflation or slight withdrawal of a distally positioned catheter to a more proximal PA location may alleviate this problem.

Damping of the PAW pressure produces the same type of rounded-out appearance as with the PA pressure with lack of defined *a* or *v* waves. The balloon should be deflated before the catheter is aspirated and then gently flushed. Never flush in the PAW position.

Occasionally a mixed PA/PAW pressure is obtained due to incomplete wedging of the catheter tip. Frequently observed waveform changes are directly related to respirations, with a PA pressure observed during expiration and a PAW pressure observed during inspiration. In this circumstance, slight advancement of the catheter is necessary to obtain an accurate PAW pressure.

The PAW mean pressure should be lower than the PA mean pressure, and a noticeable fall in pressure should occur as the balloon is inflated. Similarly, there should be an abrupt rise in pressure as the balloon is deflated. If the PAW pressure appears to be *higher* than the PA pressure, it is likely that the catheter tip is not in a zone 3 position, and, thus, is sensing elevated alveolar or airway pressure. Such a PAW pressure is not accurate or reflective of the LV end-diastolic pressure.

Frequently, direct LA pressures are measured via a small catheter placed in the left atrium at the time of open heart surgery. Since the PAW pressure is an indirect measurement of LA pressure, both the contour and the value of the LA pressure are the same as the PAW pressure. The LA *a* wave, produced by LA systole, is followed by the *x* descent, a decline in pressure due to atrial relaxation. The *c* wave is produced by closure of the mitral valve leaflets and may or may not be evident in the LA waveform. The *v* wave results from filling of the left atrium and bulging back of the mitral valve during ventricular systole. This is followed by the *y* descent, reflecting a decrease in LA volume during passive filling of the LV. The delay between electrical and mechanical events that one sees in the PAW pressure is less apparent with the direct LA pressure, that is, the LA *a* wave more immediately follows the P wave of the ECG.

Normal values for the LA pressure are a mean pressure of 4 to 12 mm Hg.

Although the PAW pressure is commonly used as a reflection of the LVedp, its limitations must be appreciated. Situations in which the PAW pressure *does not* equal or approximate the LVedp include:

1. Mitral stenosis
2. LA myxoma
3. Pulmonary venous obstruction
4. Decreased ventricular compliance
5. Increased pleural pressure
6. Placement of the catheter tip in a nondependent zone of the lung.

The possibility of such conditions affecting the PAW pressure measurement must be assessed before clinically interpreting an elevated PAW pressure. An elevated PAW pressure does not always mean the LVed pressure or volume is elevated. It could be a result of increased surrounding pleural pressure, or a noncompliant ventricle, or interruption of the fluid column between the catheter tip and the left atrium.

EXAMPLES

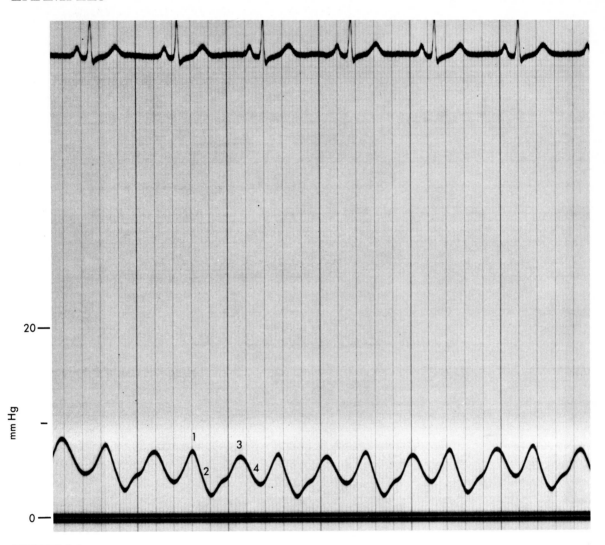

FIGURE 4-1

ANALYSIS

Rhythm: NSR

Pressure(s): PAW

Waveform characteristics and measurements:

1.	*a* Wave	;	8	mm Hg
2.	*x* Descent	;		mm Hg
3.	*v* Wave	;	8	mm Hg
4.	*y* Descent	;		mm Hg
5.	Mean	;	5	mm Hg
6.		;		mm Hg
7.		;		mm Hg

Suspected abnormality/diagnosis: Normal PAW pressure

Comments: Note the lack of respiratory variation seen when the patient momentarily suspends respirations at the end of expiration.

61

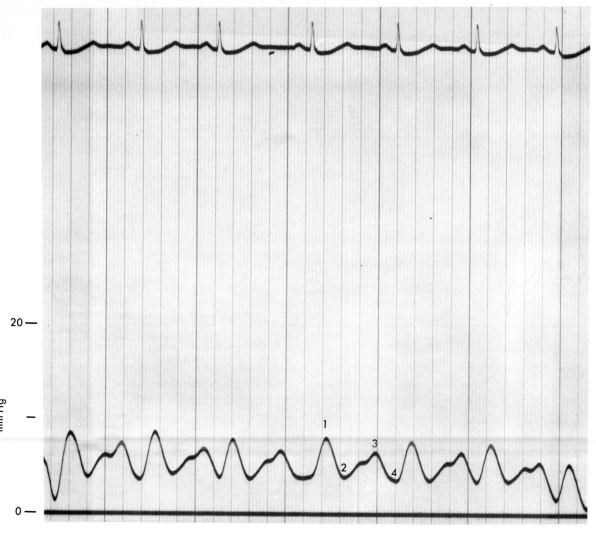

FIGURE 4-2

ANALYSIS

Rhythm: NSR

Pressure(s): PAW

Waveform characteristics and measurements:

1.	*a* Wave	;	8	mm Hg
2.	*x* Descent	;		mm Hg
3.	*v* Wave	;	7	mm Hg
4.	*y* Descent	;		mm Hg
5.		;		mm Hg
6.		;		mm Hg
7.		;		mm Hg

Suspected abnormality/diagnosis: Normal PAW pressure

Comments:

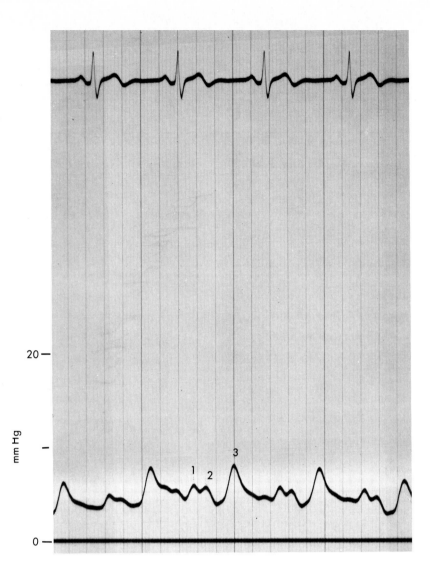

FIGURE 4-3

ANALYSIS

Rhythm: NSR

Pressure(s): PAW

Waveform characteristics and measurements:

1.	*a* Wave	;	5	mm Hg
2.	*c* Wave	;		mm Hg
3.	*v* Wave	;	8	mm Hg
4.	Mean	;	6	mm Hg
5.		;		mm Hg
6.		;		mm Hg
7.		;		mm Hg

Suspected abnormality/diagnosis: Normal or hypovolemia

Comments: This PAW pressure tracing falls within the normal range (mean of 6 mm Hg), albeit on the low side. If, however, this patient had evidence of a low cardiac output, this PAW pressure value would be considered too low, and this patient would warrant careful volume administration.

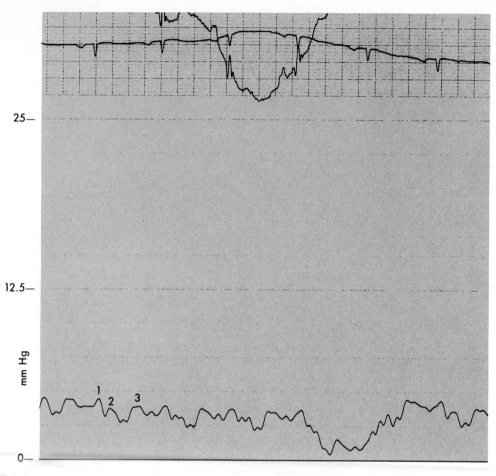

FIGURE 4-4

ANALYSIS

Rhythm: NSR

Pressure(s): PAW

Waveform characteristics and measurements:

1.	_a_ Wave	;	4	mm Hg
2.	_c_ Wave	;		mm Hg
3.	_v_ Wave	;	4	mm Hg
4.	Mean	;	3	mm Hg
5.		;		mm Hg
6.		;		mm Hg
7.		;		mm Hg

Suspected abnormality/diagnosis: Hypovolemia

Comments: This low PAW pressure suggests hypovolemia and the need for volume administration.

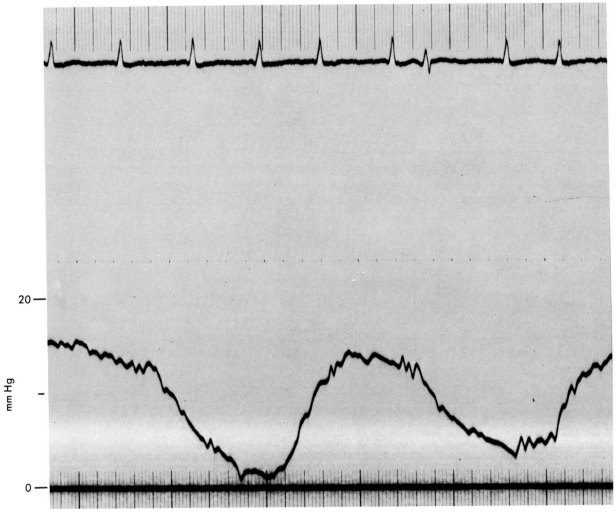

FIGURE 4-5

ANALYSIS

Rhythm: Atrial fibrillation

Pressure(s): PAW

Waveform characteristics and measurements:

1. _____ Mean _____ ; _____ 12 _____ mm Hg
2. _____ ; _____ mm Hg
3. _____ ; _____ mm Hg
4. _____ ; _____ mm Hg
5. _____ ; _____ mm Hg
6. _____ ; _____ mm Hg
7. _____ ; _____ mm Hg

Suspected abnormality/diagnosis: Normal PAW pressure

Comments: This PAW is damped with marked respiratory variation, making accurate waveform identification difficult.

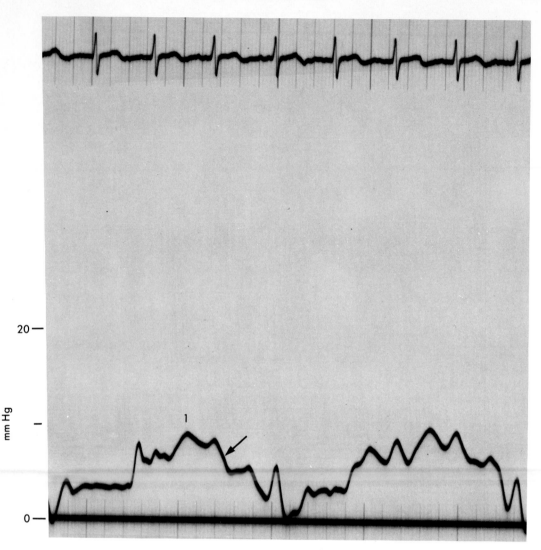

FIGURE 4-6

ANALYSIS

Rhythm: Regular supraventricular tachycardia

Pressure(s): PAW

Waveform characteristics and measurements:

1.	*v* Wave	;	6	mm Hg
2.	Mean	;	6	mm Hg
3.		;		mm Hg
4.		;		mm Hg
5.		;		mm Hg
6.		;		mm Hg
7.		;		mm Hg

Suspected abnormality/diagnosis: Normal or hypovolemia

Comments: Note normal respiratory variation with a mean pressure of approximately 6 mm Hg at end-expiration *(arrow).*

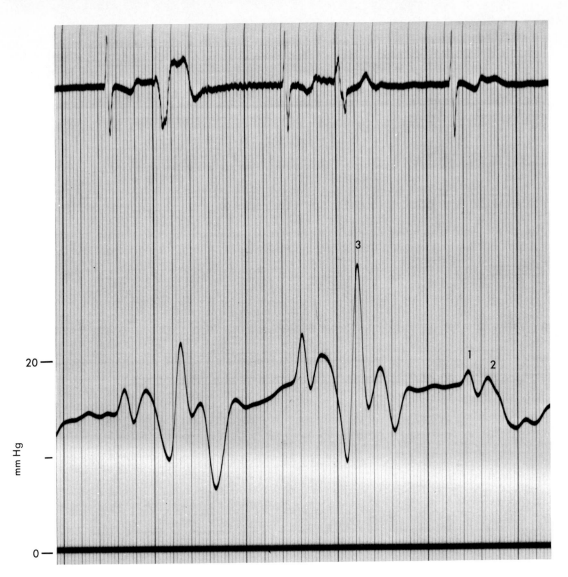

FIGURE 4-7

ANALYSIS

Rhythm: Supraventricular with PVCs

Pressure(s): PAW

Waveform characteristics and measurements:

1.	*c* Wave	;	mm Hg
2.	*v* Wave	; 18	mm Hg
3.	Early *v* wave 2° PVC	; 25-30	mm Hg
4.	Mean	; 15	mm Hg
5.		;	mm Hg
6.		;	mm Hg
7.		;	mm Hg

Suspected abnormality/diagnosis: High normal PAW pressure

Comments: Absent *a* waves are due to the supraventricular rhythm. The prominent and elevated *v* wave following the premature ventricular contraction reflects an increase in LA volume when ventricular systole occurs early while the mitral valve is open.

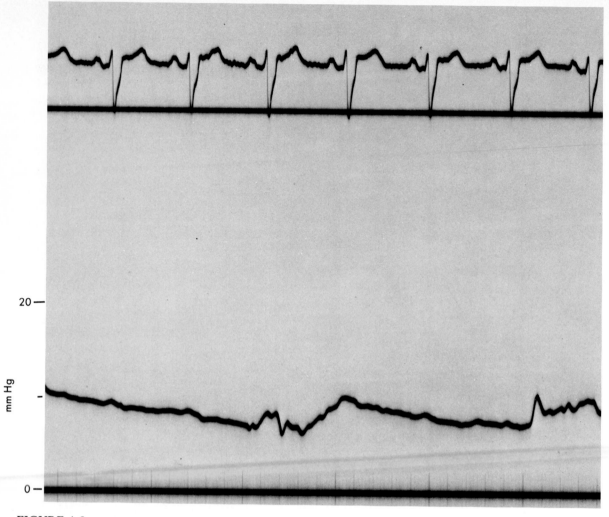

FIGURE 4-8

ANALYSIS

Rhythm: NSR

Pressure(s): (?) PAW

Waveform characteristics and measurements:

1. _____ ; _____ mm Hg
2. _____ ; _____ mm Hg
3. _____ ; _____ mm Hg
4. _____ ; _____ mm Hg
5. _____ ; _____ mm Hg
6. _____ ; _____ mm Hg
7. _____ ; _____ mm Hg

Suspected abnormality/diagnosis: Overwedged pressure

Comments: Overwedging occurs when the balloon of the catheter is either inflated with an excessive amount of air for the size vessel in which the catheter is positioned, or is eccentrically inflated allowing the balloon to cover some or all of the distal lumen. Characteristically, the pressure appears to angle either upward or downward, as in this case. Careful monitoring of the pressure waveforms during balloon inflation, with immediate cessation of inflation when a PAW waveform is obtained, can prevent this problem. If a PAW pressure waveform appears after inflation of only a small amount of air, the catheter may have advanced too far distally into a smaller caliber vessel and should be withdrawn slightly.

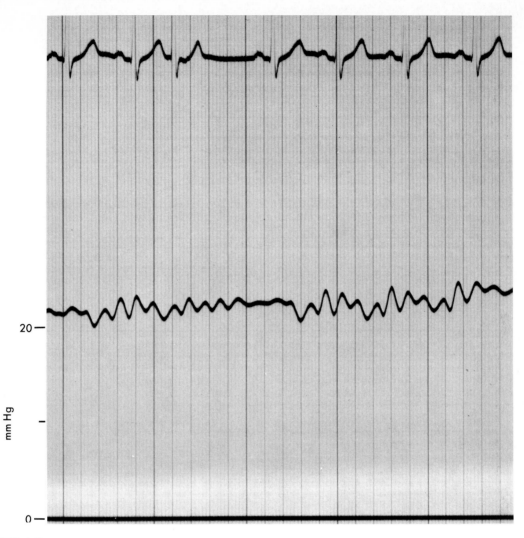

20 —

-

mm Hg

0 —

FIGURE 4-9

ANALYSIS

Rhythm: NSR with PNB

Pressure(s): PAW

Waveform characteristics and measurements:

1. _____ Mean _____ ; _____ 24 _____ mm Hg
2. _____ ; _____ mm Hg
3. _____ ; _____ mm Hg
4. _____ ; _____ mm Hg
5. _____ ; _____ mm Hg
6. _____ ; _____ mm Hg
7. _____ ; _____ mm Hg

Suspected abnormality/diagnosis: Overinflation of the balloon

Comments: This damped PAW pressure tracing is the result of overinflation of the balloon of the Swan-Ganz catheter. Although the amount of air injected may not exceed the manufacturer's recommendation, it may exceed the size of the vessel the catheter tip lies in. This could also reflect catheter positioning in zone 1 or 2 in which the microvasculature is not maintained open during balloon inflation.

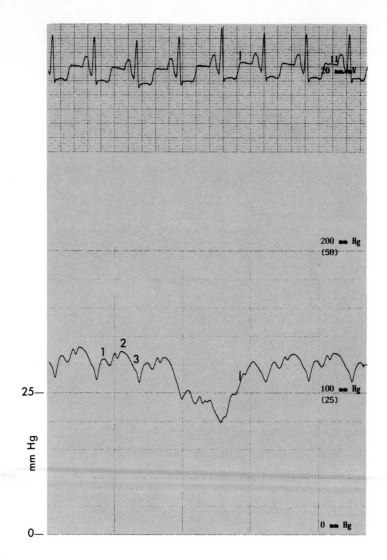

FIGURE 4-10

ANALYSIS

Rhythm: NSR

Pressure(s): PAW

Waveform characteristics and measurements:

1.	*a* Wave	;	30	mm Hg
2.	*v* Wave	;	32	mm Hg
3.	*y* Descent	;		mm Hg
4.	Mean	;	28	mm Hg
5.		;		mm Hg
6.		;		mm Hg
7.		;		mm Hg

Suspected abnormality/diagnosis: Mitral stenosis

Comments: Both the *a* and *v* waves of this PAW pressure are elevated due to stenosis of the mitral valve. Note the slow *y* descent reflecting reduced rate of atrial emptying because of the stenotic mitral valve.

70

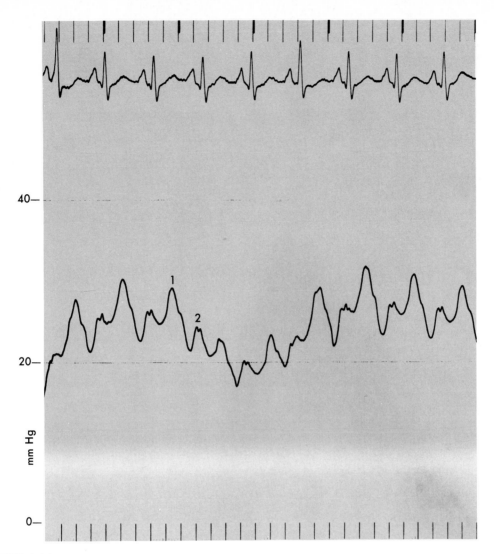

FIGURE 4-11

ANALYSIS

Rhythm: NSR

Pressure(s): PAW

Waveform characteristics and measurements:

1.	*a* Wave	; 30	mm Hg
2.	*v* Wave	; 24	mm Hg
3.	Mean	; 25	mm Hg
4.		;	mm Hg
5.		;	mm Hg
6.		;	mm Hg
7.		;	mm Hg

Suspected abnormality/diagnosis: LV failure

Comments: The dominant, elevated *a* wave of this PAW tracing is secondary to LV hypertrophy with decreased ventricular compliance.

71

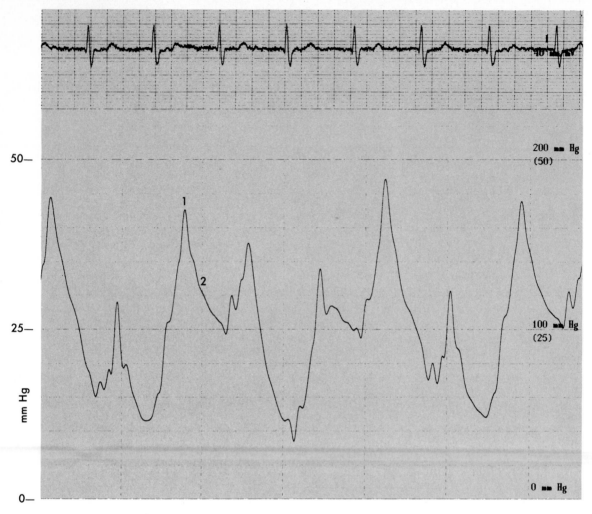

FIGURE 4-12

ANALYSIS

Rhythm: Atrial fibrillation

Pressure(s): PAW

Waveform characteristics and measurements:

1.	*v* Wave	; 35	mm Hg
2.	*y* Descent	;	mm Hg
3.		;	mm Hg
4.		;	mm Hg
5.		;	mm Hg
6.		;	mm Hg
7.		;	mm Hg

Suspected abnormality/diagnosis: Mitral regurgitation

Comments: The very early appearance of the *v* wave following the ECG T wave, as well as its elevation, indicate severe mitral regurgitation.

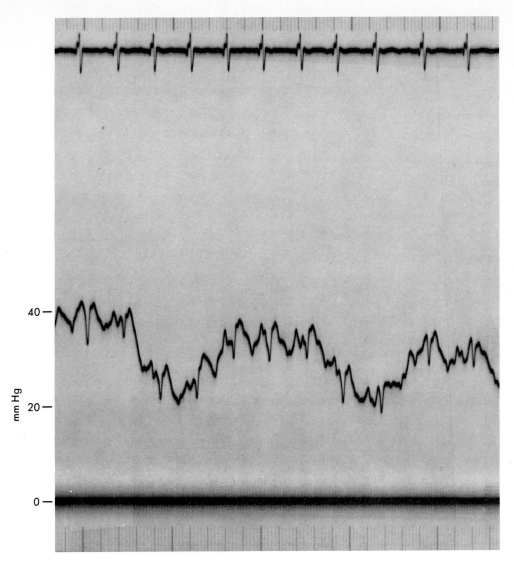

FIGURE 4-13

ANALYSIS

Rhythm: Rapid atrial fibrillation

Pressure(s): PAW

Waveform characteristics and measurements:

1.	Mean	; 30	mm Hg
2.		;	mm Hg
3.		;	mm Hg
4.		;	mm Hg
5.		;	mm Hg
6.		;	mm Hg
7.		;	mm Hg

Suspected abnormality/diagnosis: CHF

Comments: There are no *a* waves in this PAW tracing because of atrial fibrillation. The rapid heart rate and numerous fibrillatory waves make identification of the *v* wave difficult. In this case, the mean PAW pressure at end-expiration is used to reflect LVedp.

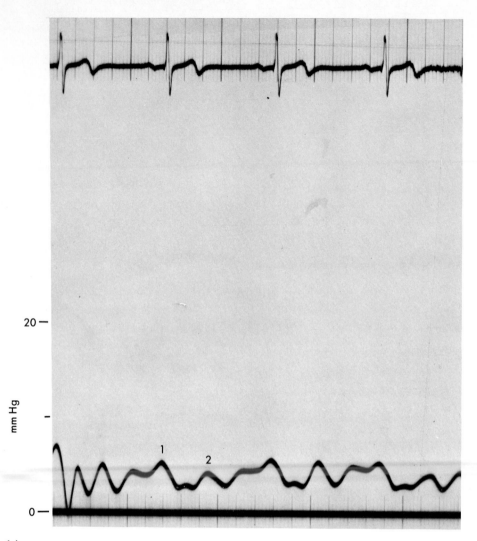

FIGURE 4-14

ANALYSIS

Rhythm: NSR

Pressure(s): PAW

Waveform characteristics and measurements:

1.	*a* Wave	;	5	mm Hg
2.	*v* Wave	;	5	mm Hg
3.	Mean	;	5	mm Hg
4.		;		mm Hg
5.		;		mm Hg
6.		;		mm Hg
7.		;		mm Hg

Suspected abnormality/diagnosis: Abnormally low PAW secondary to nitroprusside administration

Comments: Nitroprusside is a balanced venous and arterial vasodilator and therefore reduces both preload and afterload. During nitroprusside administration, particular attention must be given the PAW or PAedp to prevent reduction of the preload level to that point on the Starling ventricular function curve where cardiac output falls. Commonly, administration of volume during nitroprusside therapy is necessary to maintain an adequate preload level.

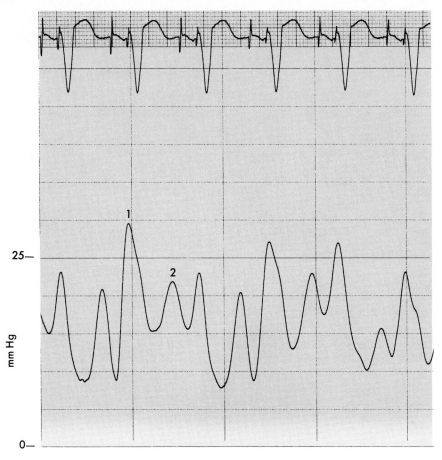

25—

mm Hg

0—

FIGURE 4-15

ANALYSIS

Rhythm: A-V sequential pacing

Pressure(s): PAW

Waveform characteristics and measurements:

1.	*a* Wave	;	26	mm Hg
2.	*v* Wave	;	22	mm Hg
3.	Mean	;	20	mm Hg
4.		;		mm Hg
5.		;		mm Hg
6.		;		mm Hg
7.		;		mm Hg

Suspected abnormality/diagnosis: LV failure

Comments: Although both the *a* and *v* wave are elevated in this PAW tracing, the slightly dominant *a* wave of 26 mm Hg suggests LV failure and decreased ventricular compliance.

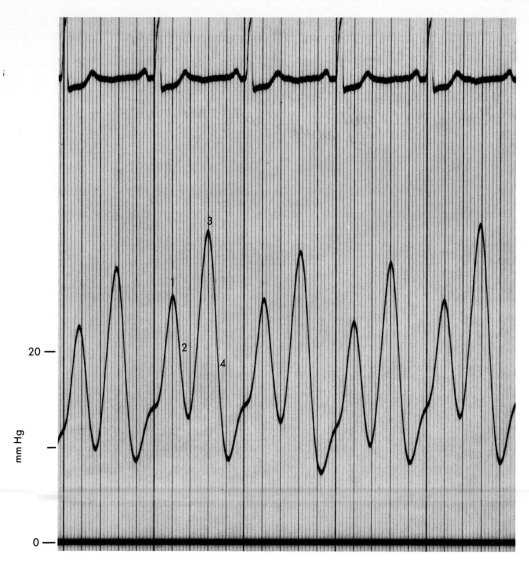

FIGURE 4-16

ANALYSIS

Rhythm: NSR

Pressure(s): PAW

Waveform characteristics and measurements:

1.	*a* Wave	;	26	mm Hg
2.	*x* Descent	;		mm Hg
3.	*v* Wave	;	32	mm Hg
4.	*y* Descent	;		mm Hg
5.		;		mm Hg
6.		;		mm Hg
7.		;		mm Hg

Suspected abnormality/diagnosis: LVH with mild mitral regurgitation

Comments: The elevated *a* wave of 26 mm Hg suggests increased resistance to LV filling, as in the case of LVH, where the ventricle becomes stiff and noncompliant. The elevated and dominant *v* wave indicates decreased LA compliance or, perhaps, mild mitral regurgitation.

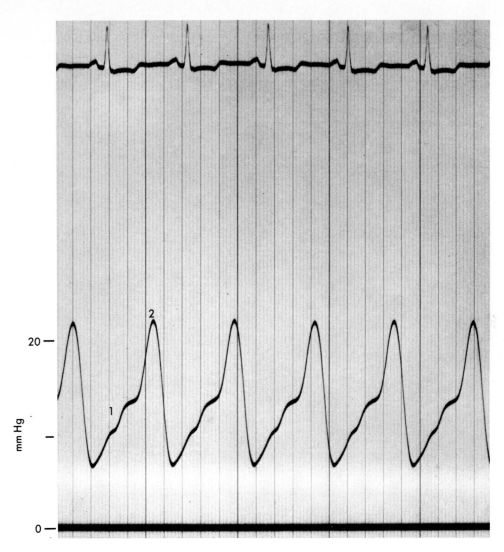

FIGURE 4-17

ANALYSIS

Rhythm: NSR

Pressure(s): PAW

Waveform characteristics and measurements:

1.	*a* Wave	;	10	mm Hg
2.	*v* Wave	;	22	mm Hg
3.		;		mm Hg
4.		;		mm Hg
5.		;		mm Hg
6.		;		mm Hg
7.		;		mm Hg

Suspected abnormality/diagnosis: Mild mitral regurgitation or decreased LA compliance

Comments: The elevated, dominant *v* wave due to mitral regurgitation and blood flow into the left atrium during ventricular systole almost obscures the *a* wave in this PAW pressure waveform. However, the low value of the *a* wave (10 mm Hg) indicates that the left ventricle is performing well without evidence of LV failure at this time.

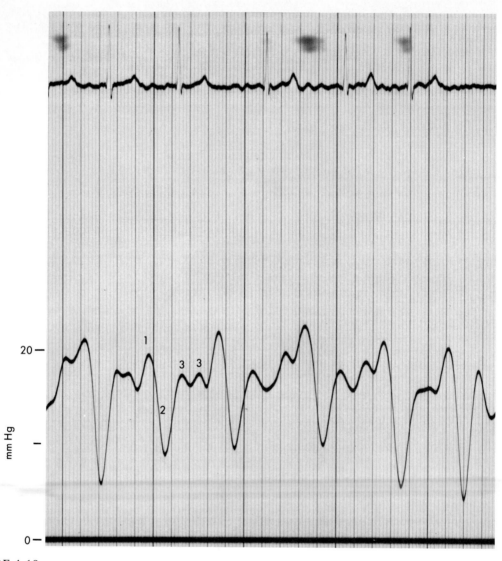

FIGURE 4-18

ANALYSIS

Rhythm: Atrial fibrillation

Pressure(s): PAW

Waveform characteristics and measurements:

1.	v Wave	; 25	mm Hg
2.	y Descent	;	mm Hg
3.	Possible fibrillation waves	;	mm Hg
4.		;	mm Hg
5.		;	mm Hg
6.		;	mm Hg
7.		;	mm Hg

Suspected abnormality/diagnosis: CHF, possible mitral regurgitation

Comments: The elevated v wave and rapid y descent are suggestive of mild mitral regurgitation.

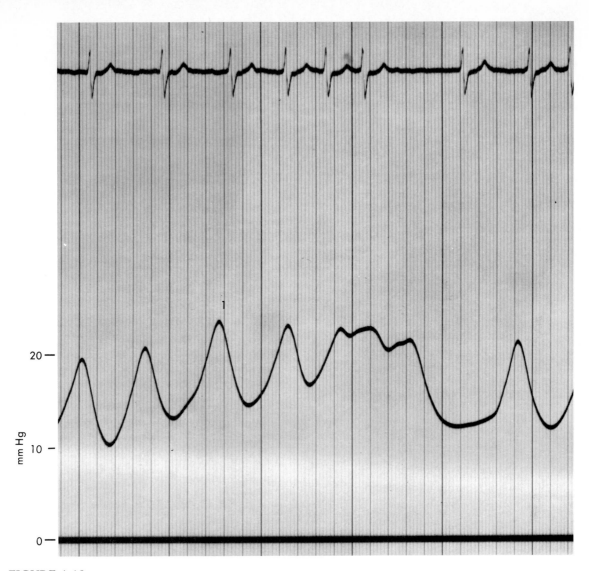

FIGURE 4-19

ANALYSIS

Rhythm: Atrial fibrillation

Pressure(s): PAW

Waveform characteristics and measurements:

1.	v Wave	; 22	mm Hg
2.	Mean	; 15	mm Hg
3.		;	mm Hg
4.		;	mm Hg
5.		;	mm Hg
6.		;	mm Hg
7.		;	mm Hg

Suspected abnormality/diagnosis: Mild to moderate mitral regurgitation

Comments: Note the effect of a three-beat run of tachycardia on the PAW pressure contour. This is due to the reduction in LV filling time, resulting in increased LA volume throughout the cardiac cycle; consequently, LA pressure remains elevated.

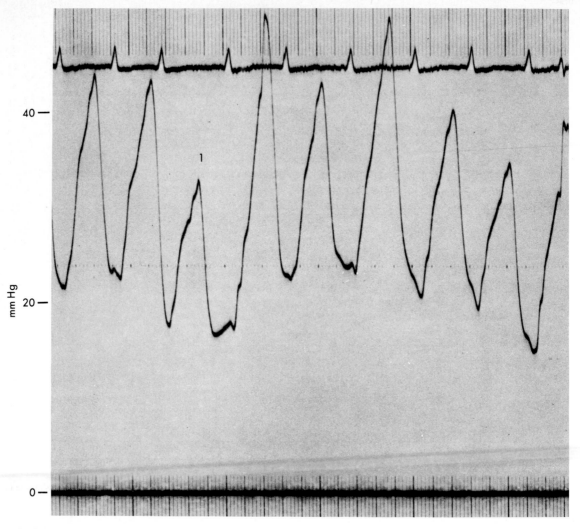

FIGURE 4-20

ANALYSIS

Rhythm: Atrial fibrillation

Pressure(s): PAW

Waveform characteristics and measurements:

1.	*v* Wave	; 48	mm Hg
2.		;	mm Hg
3.		;	mm Hg
4.		;	mm Hg
5.		;	mm Hg
6.		;	mm Hg
7.		;	mm Hg

Suspected abnormality/diagnosis: Severe mitral regurgitation

Comments: A single *v* wave is seen corresponding with each T wave. The lack of *a* waves is due to atrial fibrillation. The elevated and dominant *v* wave is caused by mitral regurgitation with retrograde flow of blood into the left atrium during ventricular systole. Note the variation in the height of the *v* waves dependent on the RR interval and duration of LV filling. The third *v* wave is only about 30 mm Hg because of the short preceding RR interval and decreased filling of the LV resulting in decreased regurgitant volume. The fourth *v* wave, on the other hand, is markedly higher (52 mm Hg) because of the longer preceding RR interval and filling time of the LV.

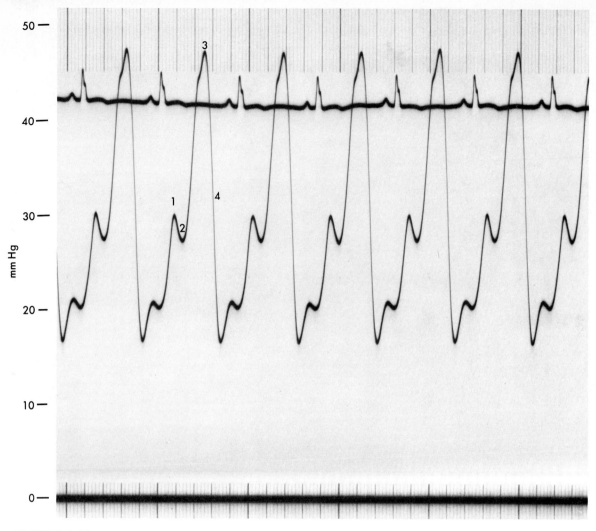

FIGURE 4-21

ANALYSIS

Rhythm: NSR

Pressure(s): PAW

Waveform characteristics and measurements:

1.	*a* Wave	;	30	mm Hg
2.	*x* Descent	;		mm Hg
3.	*v* Wave	;	41	mm Hg
4.	*y* Descent	;		mm Hg
5.		;		mm Hg
6.		;		mm Hg
7.		;		mm Hg

Suspected abnormality/diagnosis: LV failure with mitral regurgitation

Comments: The elevated and dominant *v* wave indicates mitral regurgitation, whereas the elevated *a* wave indicates LV failure. In this situation it is the PAW *a* wave that reflects LVedp, not the PAW mean pressure.

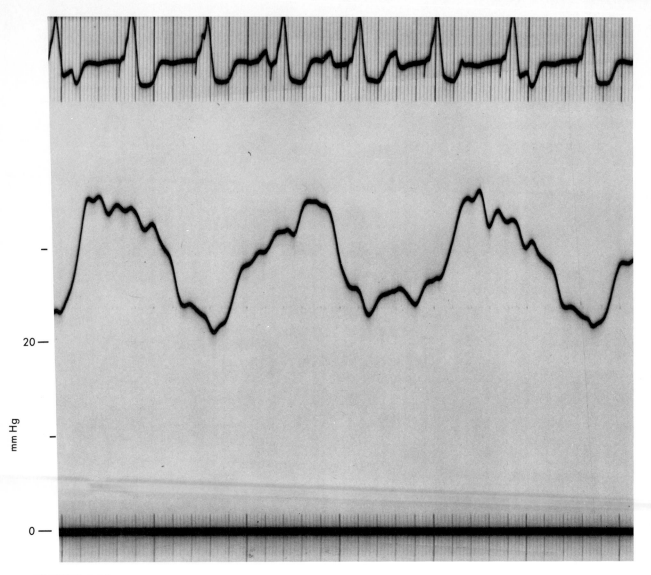

FIGURE 4-22

ANALYSIS

Rhythm: Paced (Note the pacemaker spikes and P waves throughout the ECG.)

Pressure(s): PAW

Waveform characteristics and measurements:

1. _____Mean_____ ; _____28_____ mm Hg
2. _____ ; _____ mm Hg
3. _____ ; _____ mm Hg
4. _____ ; _____ mm Hg
5. _____ ; _____ mm Hg
6. _____ ; _____ mm Hg
7. _____ ; _____ mm Hg

Suspected abnormality/diagnosis: Acute pulmonary edema

Comments: Such marked respiratory variation is commonly seen with acute pulmonary edema or chronic obstructive pulmonary disease (COPD). The mean pressure measured at end-expiration averages approximately 28 mm Hg.

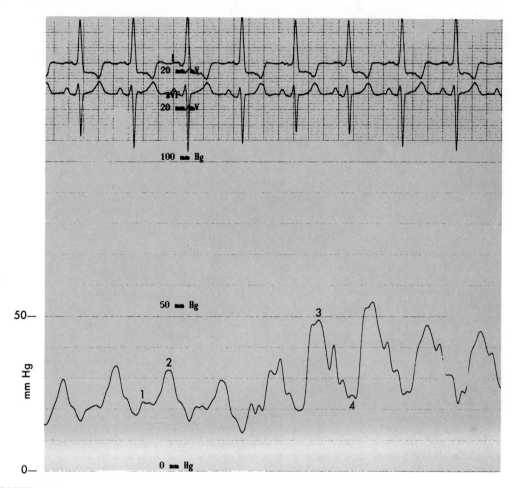

FIGURE 4-23

ANALYSIS

Rhythm: NSR

Pressure(s): PAW to PA

Waveform characteristics and measurements:

1.	PAW *a* wave	;	22	mm Hg
2.	PAW *v* wave	;	34	mm Hg
3.	PA systolic	;	48	mm Hg
4.	PA diastolic	;	24	mm Hg
5.		;		mm Hg
6.		;		mm Hg
7.		;		mm Hg

Suspected abnormality/diagnosis: Pulmonary hypertension secondary to LV failure

Comments: The elevated PAW *a* wave of 22 mm Hg suggests LV failure while the dominant and elevated *v* wave reflects mitral regurgitation. Note the similarity between the PA end-diastolic and PAW *a* wave.

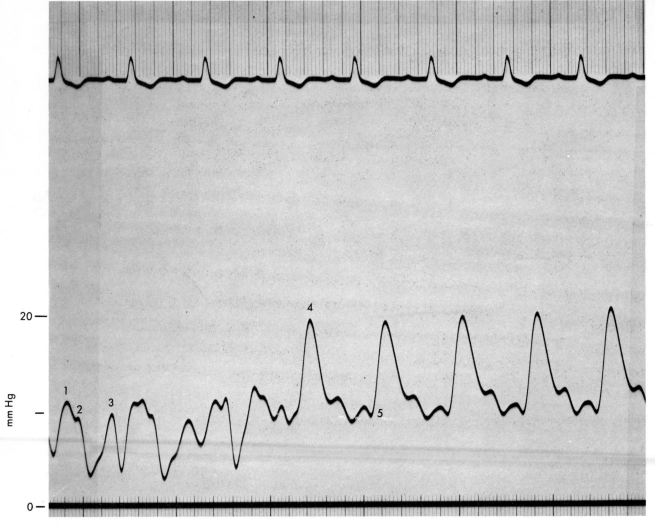

FIGURE 4-24

ANALYSIS

Rhythm: NSR

Pressure(s): PAW to PA

Waveform characteristics and measurements:

1.	PAW *a* wave	;	11	mm Hg
2.	PAW *c* wave	;		mm Hg
3.	PAW *v* wave	;	9	mm Hg
4.	PA systolic	;	20	mm Hg
5.	PA end-diastolic	;	10	mm Hg
6.		;		mm Hg
7.		;		mm Hg

Suspected abnormality/diagnosis: PAW and PA pressures

Comments: Note the correlation between the mean PAW and PAedp, obviating the need to measure the PAW pressure.

84

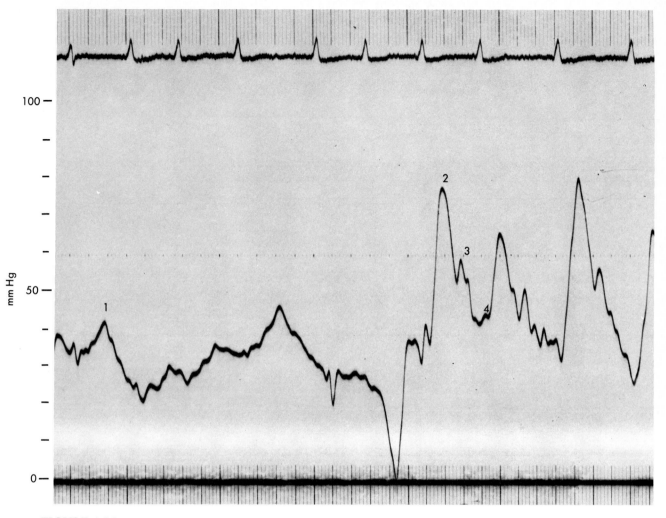

FIGURE 4-25

ANALYSIS

Rhythm: Atrial fibrillation

Pressure(s): PAW to PA

Waveform characteristics and measurements:

1.	PAW *v* wave	;	34	mm Hg
2.	PA systolic	;	70	mm Hg
3.	Dicrotic notch	;		mm Hg
4.	PA end-diastolic	;	32	mm Hg
5.		;		mm Hg
6.		;		mm Hg
7.		;		mm Hg

Suspected abnormality/diagnosis: Pulmonary hypertension secondary to severe CHF

Comments: Because of atrial fibrillation, there is only a *v* wave present in this PAW pressure waveform. Although there is considerable respiratory variation, the PAW pressure averages approximately 34 mm Hg, indicating severe CHF. Note the close correlation between the PAW mean and the PAedp.

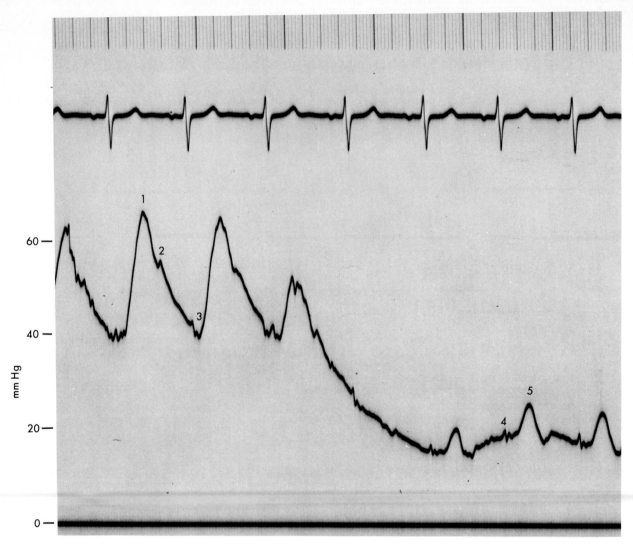

FIGURE 4-26

ANALYSIS

Rhythm: NSR

Pressure(s): PA to PAW

Waveform characteristics and measurements:

#			Value	
1.	PA systolic	;	65	mm Hg
2.	Dicrotic notch	;		mm Hg
3.	PA end-diastolic	;	40	mm Hg
4.	PAW *a* wave	;	18	mm Hg
5.	PAW *v* wave	;	21	mm Hg
6.		;		mm Hg
7.		;		mm Hg

Suspected abnormality/diagnosis: Pulmonary hypertension secondary to COPD with mild LV failure

Comments: Note the disparity between the PAedp and PAW pressure. This pulmonary hypertension is due to chronic lung disease and, therefore does not reflect the LVedp. The PAW pressure, however, does reflect the LVedp and reveals mild LV failure (18 mm Hg) and perhaps a very small amount of mitral regurgitation secondary to LV dilatation.

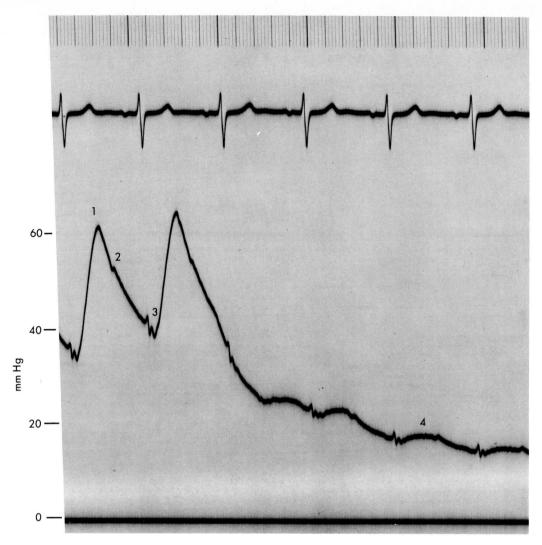

FIGURE 4-27

ANALYSIS

Rhythm: NSR

Pressure(s): PA to PAW

Waveform characteristics and measurements:

1.	PA systolic	;	60	mm Hg
2.	Dicrotic notch	;		mm Hg
3.	PA end-diastolic	;	37	mm Hg
4.	PAW mean	;	18	mm Hg
5.		;		mm Hg
6.		;		mm Hg
7.		;		mm Hg

Suspected abnormality/diagnosis: Pulmonary hypertension secondary to COPD with mild LV failure

Comments: These pressures are recorded from the same patient as in Figure 4-26; however, these pressure waveforms are damped, making the accuracy of the pressure values questionable. Note particularly the lack of identifiable waves in the PAW pressure tracing. This catheter should be aspirated and flushed in the PA position before the recording of new pressures.

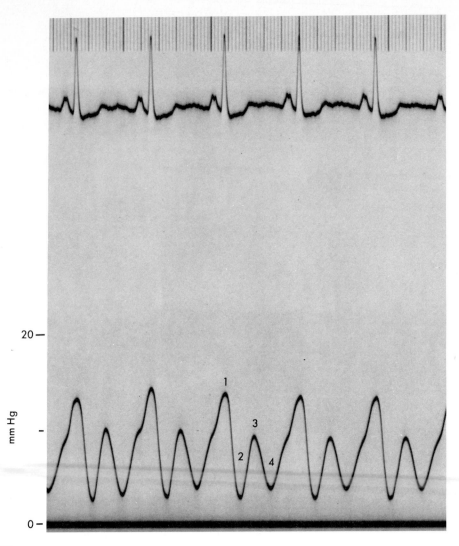

FIGURE 4-28

ANALYSIS

Rhythm: NSR

Pressure(s): LA

Waveform characteristics and measurements:

1.	*a* Wave	;	14	mm Hg
2.	*x* Descent	;		mm Hg
3.	*v* Wave	;	10	mm Hg
4.	Mean	;	9	mm Hg
5.		;		mm Hg
6.		;		mm Hg
7.		;		mm Hg

Suspected abnormality/diagnosis: Normal LA pressure

Comments: Note the lack of respiratory response due to momentarily suspended respirations.

88

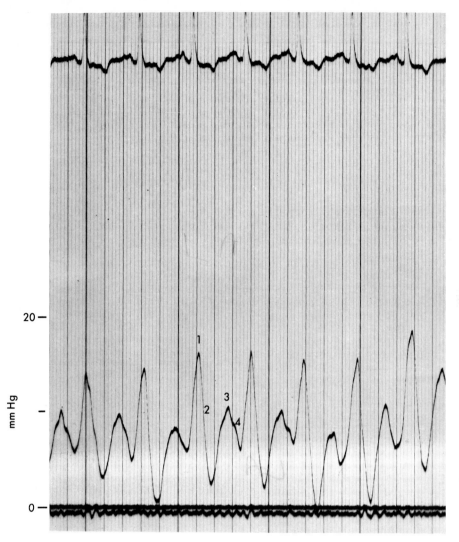

FIGURE 4-29

ANALYSIS

Rhythm: Sinus tachycardia

Pressure(s): LA

Waveform characteristics and measurements:

1.	*a* Wave	;	16	mm Hg
2.	*x* Descent	;		mm Hg
3.	*v* Wave	;	10	mm Hg
4.	*y* Descent	;		mm Hg
5.		;		mm Hg
6.		;		mm Hg
7.		;		mm Hg

Suspected abnormality/diagnosis: LVH

Comments: The values of this LA pressure are normal, but the prominent *a* wave with rapid *x* descent suggests a somewhat stiff, hypertrophic LV.

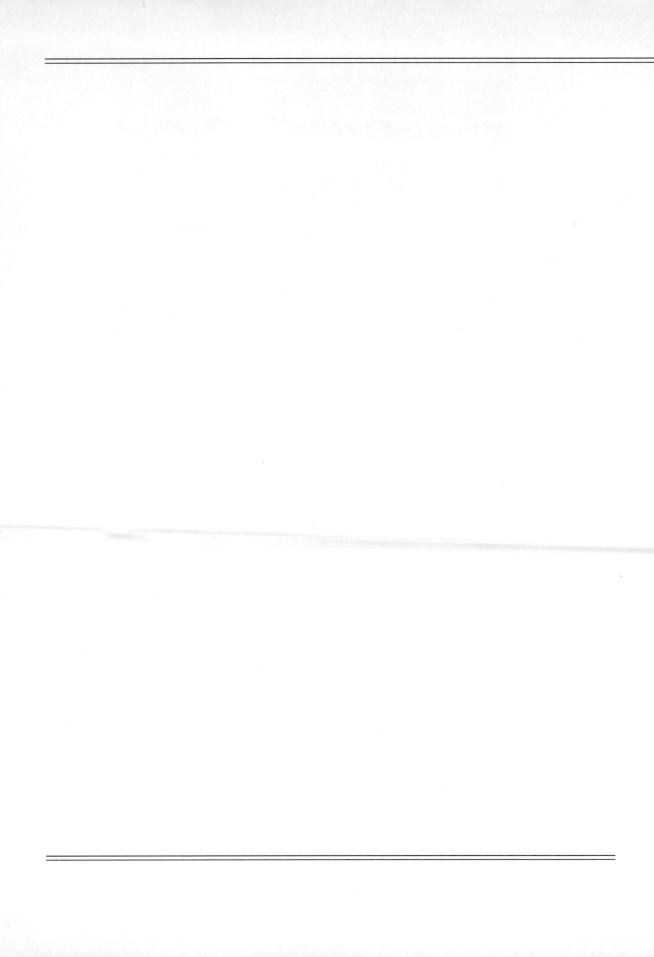

Chapter 5

Arterial Pressures

Physiology and Morphology

The arterial pressure waveform resembles the PA pressure waveform in contour, since the same physiologic events occur on the left side of the heart as on the right side of the heart. The value, however, is normally six times greater on the left side of the heart. The arterial pressure is divided into two phases: systole and diastole. Aterial systole begins with the opening of the aortic valve and rapid ejection of blood into the aorta. This is followed by runoff of blood from the proximal aorta to the peripheral arteries. On the arterial pressure waveform this is seen as a sharp rise in pressure followed by a decline in pressure. As the pressure falls, the aortic valve snaps shut, causing a small rise in arterial pressure that appears as a dip on the downslope and is termed the *dicrotic notch*. The *peak systolic pressure* (which reflects LV systolic pressure) is normally 100 to 140 mm Hg.

Diastole follows closure of the aortic valve and continues until the next systole. During this time, run-off to the peripheral arteries occurs without further flow from the LV. On the arterial pressure waveform this is seen as a gradual decrease in pressure. The lowest point of diastole (actually, end-diastole) is referred to as the *arterial diastolic pressure* and is normally 60 to 80 mm Hg.

The *mean arterial pressure (MAP)* represents the average arterial pressure during systole and diastole. Normal mean arterial pressure is 70 to 90 mm Hg. The mean pressure is dependent on both the volume of bloodflow through the vessel (cardiac output) and the elasticity or resistance of the vessels (systemic vascular resistance). This interrelation can be expressed as:

$$\text{MAP} = \text{Cardiac output} \times \text{Systemic vascular resistance}$$

The pulse pressure is the difference between the systolic and diastolic pressure and is largely reflective of the stroke volume and arterial compliance. Wide pulse pressures are associated with large stroke volumes (such as aortic regurgitation) while a narrow pulse pressure is seen in patients with low stroke volume.

The arterial pressure differs in both contour and value in various arterial locations. The systolic pressure is higher in the femoral artery than in the radial or brachial artery, by as much as 25 to 50 mm Hg. Generally, the diastolic values remain approximately the same. Additionally, the more distal the location of the arterial catheter, the sharper and later the upstroke and the less defined the dicrotic notch (Figure 5-12). The more distal from the ascending aorta, the higher the arterial pressure as a result of the summation of reflected waves with the initial wave.

ECG Correlation

The systolic arterial pressure rise occurs immediately following ventricular depolarization, that is, after the QRS complex on the ECG. Again, there may be some delay, depending on the catheter location and length of tubing used. The dicrotic notch occurs after the T wave of the ECG.

In atrial fibrillation the arterial pressure value varies considerably (Figure 5-3) depending on the RR intervals and length of time for ventricular filling. However, the normal characteristics of the arterial waveform are still present.

When a PVC occurs, ventricular systole is initiated early, before the LV has had time to fill with blood. This results in a diminished stroke volume and lowered arterial pulse pressure. Isolated PVCs are usually well compensated for by a pause and an increase in stroke volume and arterial pressure with the succeeding contraction. Runs of PVCs, however, can be devastating, since there is virtually no opportunity for LV filling and, therefore stroke volume and arterial pressure fall precipitously (Figure 5-9).

Abnormal Findings

In addition to undergoing changes as it travels distally, the pulse wave of the arterial system can exhibit changes related to specific underlying pathology.

The arterial pressure is elevated in the following conditions:
1. Systemic hypertension
2. Arteriosclerosis
3. Aortic insufficiency

The arterial pressure waveform with aortic insufficiency classically reveals a wide pulse pressure with an elevated systolic pressure and a lowered diastolic pressure (Figure 5-6). This is due to rapid ejection of a large stroke volume (the normal stroke volume plus the regurgitant volume), with regurgitation of blood across the incompetent aortic valve during diastole. Additionally, the dicrotic notch on the downslope of the arterial pressure is usually absent.

Additionally, certain drugs, including vasopressors and certain positive inotropic agents, can markedly increase arterial pressure by increasing systemic vascular resistance and/or increasing cardiac output.

The arterial pressure may be abnormally low in the following conditions:
1. Low cardiac output
2. Aortic stenosis
3. Arrhythmias

Certain drugs, including vasodilators and certain calcium antagonists, can also decrease arterial blood pressure by decreasing systemic vascular resistance.

The contour of the arterial pressure waveform with low cardiac output or even the state of shock is normal, but the systolic value is abnormally low and the pulse pressure is narrow due to the small stroke volume ejected each beat.

Both the contour and the value of the arterial pressure are altered with aortic stenosis. Because of the increased resistance to ejection of blood through the narrowed aortic valve orifice, the upstroke of the arterial pressure waveform is slow and appears to rise at an angle rather than straight up. Often the dicrotic notch is not well defined and may appear as a "bend" on the downslope of the arterial pressure waveform. This is caused by the stiff closing movement of diseased aortic valve leaflets, which does not produce a rise in pressure. The value of the arterial pressure is low with a narrow pulse pressure, indicating a low stroke volume. It should be mentioned here that the contour of a damped arterial waveform closely resembles the arterial waveform of aortic stenosis.

Other distinct pathological changes in the configuration of the arterial pressure waveform include:

1. Pulsus bisferiens
2. Pulsus alternans
3. Pulsus paradoxus

Pulsus bisferiens describes an arterial pulse with two distinct systolic peaks (Figure 5-13). This characteristic feature may be found in patients with aortic regurgitation or, more commonly, hypertrophic cardiomyopathy. The first peak is produced by rapid, forceful ejection of blood into the aorta. The pressure then declines slightly (in hypertrophic cardiomyopathy this is because of severe obstruction during midsystole) and is followed by a smaller pressure rise produced by continued ventricular contraction.

Pulsus alternans refers to a regular, alternating pattern of changes in pressure pulse amplitude, with every other pulse being slightly greater than the previous one (Figure 5-14). Generally, it is a result of alternating ventricular contractility and subsequent stroke volume, and it occurs commonly in patients with severe LV failure. Pulsus alternans also can occur transiently following temporary arrhythmic episodes.

Pulsus paradoxus was first described by Kussmaul as a paradoxical disappearance of peripheral arterial pulsations during inspiration despite continued regular heart beats. When the systolic arterial pressure declines more than 10 mm Hg during normal spontaneous inspiration, pulsus paradoxus is said to exist (Figure 5-11). Pulsus paradoxus classically is seen in cases of cardiac tamponade (about 70% to 80%), but also can be seen in patients with obstructed airway disease and, less commonly, in those with hypovolemic shock and pulmonary embolism. Reversed or positive pulsus paradoxus is a phenomenon describing an exaggerated *rise* in systolic arterial pressure (>10 mm Hg) during inspiration in patients receiving positive pressure ventilation. This variation in systolic pressure is thought to accurately reflect hypovolemia in patients on positive pressure ventilation and usually disappears with appropriate volume therapy.

Certain drugs, including vasodilators and calcium antagonists, also can decrease arterial blood pressure by decreasing systemic vascular resistance.

Abnormalities of the arterial pressure waveform may result from mechanical causes of damping, fling, or whip or inaccurate zeroing or calibrating. Damping produces an arterial pressure waveform similar to that of aortic stenosis, that is, a slow upstroke, rounded appearance, poorly defined dicrotic notch, and narrow pulse pressure. A clot at the tip of the catheter or lodging of the catheter tip against the vessel wall is usually the cause, and gentle flushing or repositioning of the catheter tip eliminates this problem. Fling or whip in the arterial pressure waveform may be due to excessive movement of the catheter tip (Figure 5-2).

Because of the high frequency components within the arterial pulse wave, distortion caused by inadequate dynamic response characteristics of the monitoring system is the major reason for inaccuracies in direct arterial pressure monitoring. This becomes emphasized in the presence of tachycardia, which further increases the frequency response requirements of the monitoring system.

Vasodilators (including certain calcium antagonists) affect both the contour and the value of the arterial pressure waveform. The decreased systemic vascular resistance and impedance to flow during afterload reduction cause a rapid upstroke of the arterial systolic pressure, a rapid decline in systolic pressure during the shorter ejection phase, and less change in pressure during diastole (the period of resistance-reduced runoff). The value of both the systolic and diastolic pressures are often reduced, although it is possible to greatly enhance the cardiac output and thereby cause little change in the arterial pressures.

EXAMPLES

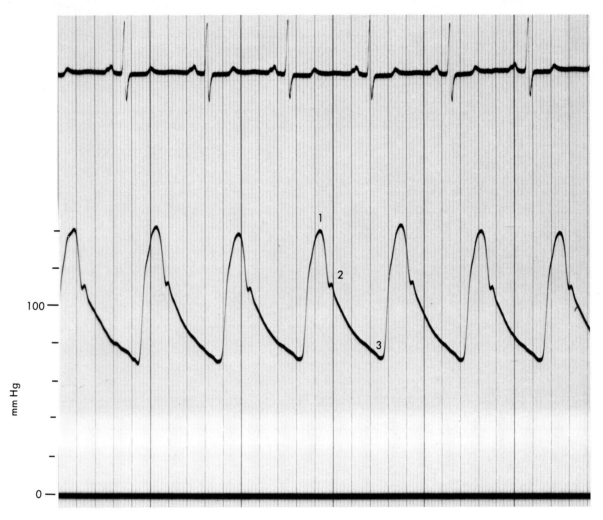

FIGURE 5-1

ANALYSIS

Rhythm: NSR

Pressure(s): Radial artery

Waveform characteristics and measurements:

1.	Arterial systolic	;	140	mm Hg
2.	Dicrotic notch	;		mm Hg
3.	Arterial end-diastolic	;	72	mm Hg
4.		;		mm Hg
5.		;		mm Hg
6.		;		mm Hg
7.		;		mm Hg

Suspected abnormality/diagnosis: Normal

Comments:

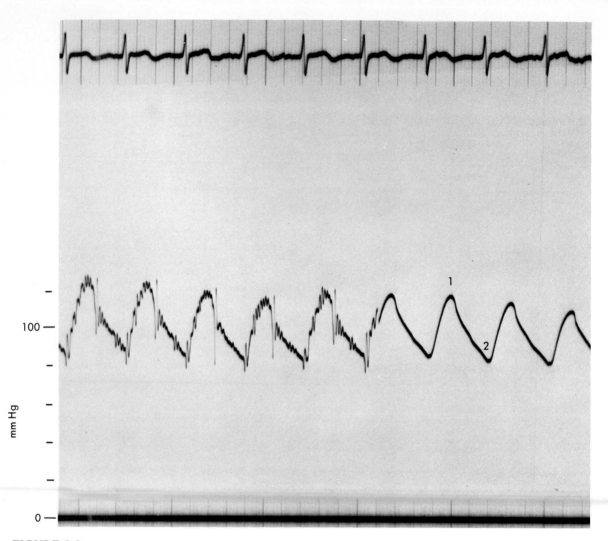

FIGURE 5-2

ANALYSIS

Rhythm: NSR

Pressure(s): Central arterial

Waveform characteristics and measurements:

1.	Arterial systolic	;	120	mm Hg
2.	Arterial end-diastolic	;	82	mm Hg
3.		;		mm Hg
4.		;		mm Hg
5.		;		mm Hg
6.		;		mm Hg
7.		;		mm Hg

Suspected abnormality/diagnosis: Normal

Comments: Note the presence of noise or fling in the first five pressure waveforms. It disappears in the last four pressure waveforms due to repositioning of the catheter tip. The contour actually becomes damped in appearance, probably due to placement of the catheter tip against the wall of the vessel. This produces a rounded-out appearance and lack of defined dicrotic notch.

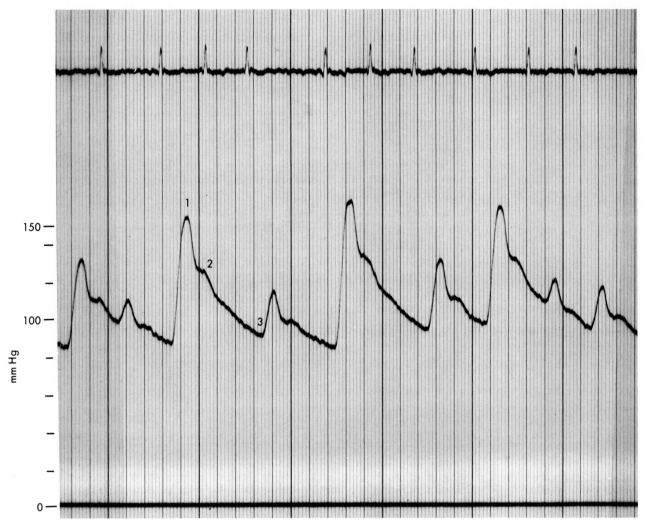

FIGURE 5-3

ANALYSIS

Rhythm: Atrial fibrillation

Pressure(s): Radial artery

Waveform characteristics and measurements:

1.	Arterial systolic	;	110-155	mm Hg
2.	Dicrotic notch	;		mm Hg
3.	Arterial end-diastolic	;	85	mm Hg
4.		;		mm Hg
5.		;		mm Hg
6.		;		mm Hg
7.		;		mm Hg

Suspected abnormality/diagnosis: Normal

Comments: Note the beat-to-beat variation in the arterial systolic pressure due to varying RR intervals with atrial fibrillation resulting in varying stroke volumes.

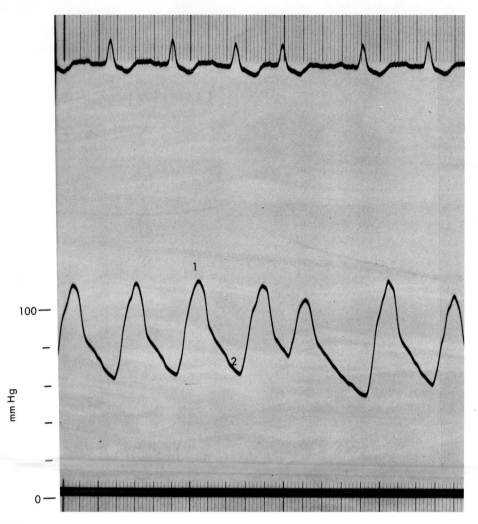

FIGURE 5-4

ANALYSIS

Rhythm: First-degree AV block with supraventricular beat
Pressure(s): Radial artery
Waveform characteristics and measurements:

1.	Arterial systolic	;	110	mm Hg
2.	Arterial end-diastolic	;	65	mm Hg
3.		;		mm Hg
4.		;		mm Hg
5.		;		mm Hg
6.		;		mm Hg
7.		;		mm Hg

Suspected abnormality/diagnosis: Normal

Comments: The damped quality of this arterial pressure waveform is evidenced by a rounded-out appearance and lack of sharp definition of the dicrotic notch. Aspiration and flushing can usually remedy this problem.

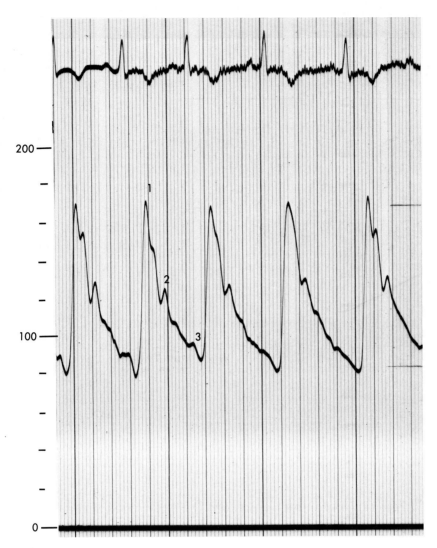

FIGURE 5-5

ANALYSIS

Rhythm: NSR

Pressure(s): Radial artery

Waveform characteristics and measurements:

1.	Arterial systolic	;	170	mm Hg
2.	Dicrotic notch	;		mm Hg
3.	Arterial end-diastolic	;	80	mm Hg
4.		;		mm Hg
5.		;		mm Hg
6.		;		mm Hg
7.		;		mm Hg

Suspected abnormality/diagnosis: Systolic hypertension

Comments:

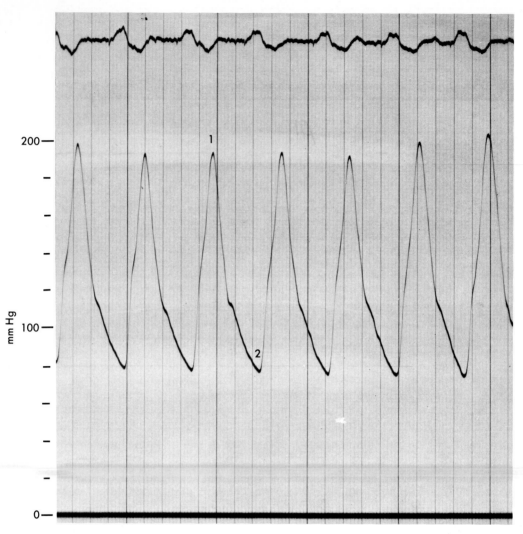

FIGURE 5-6

ANALYSIS

Rhythm: Paced

Pressure(s): Femoral artery

Waveform characteristics and measurements:

1.	Arterial systolic	; 200	mm Hg
2.	Arterial end-diastolic	; 80	mm Hg
3.		;	mm Hg
4.		;	mm Hg
5.		;	mm Hg
6.		;	mm Hg
7.		;	mm Hg

Suspected abnormality/diagnosis: Aortic regurgitation

Comments: Note the wide pulse pressure (120 mm Hg) and ill-defined dicrotic notch seen with aortic regurgitation.

100

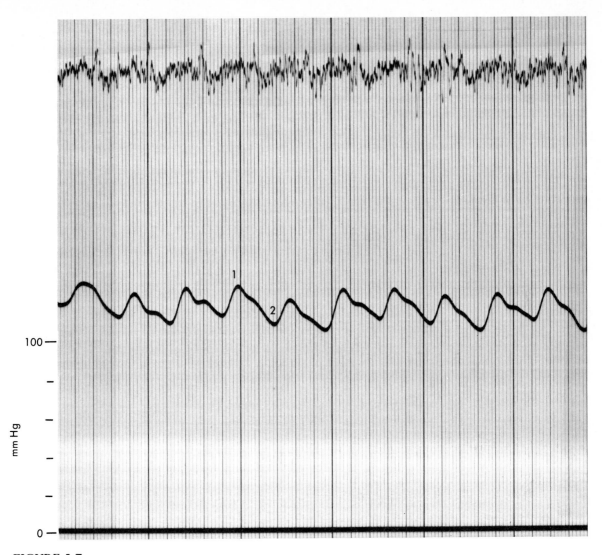

FIGURE 5-7

ANALYSIS

Rhythm: NSR (Note ECG interference.)

Pressure(s): Radial artery

Waveform characteristics and measurements:

1.	Arterial systolic	;	120	mm Hg
2.	Arterial end-diastolic	;	105	mm Hg
3.		;		mm Hg
4.		;		mm Hg
5.		;		mm Hg
6.		;		mm Hg
7.		;		mm Hg

Suspected abnormality/diagnosis: Damped pressure

Comments: This arterial pressure waveform is very damped, showing a rounded-out contour, slow upstroke, and diminished pulse pressure. Aspiration and flushing usually alleviate this problem.

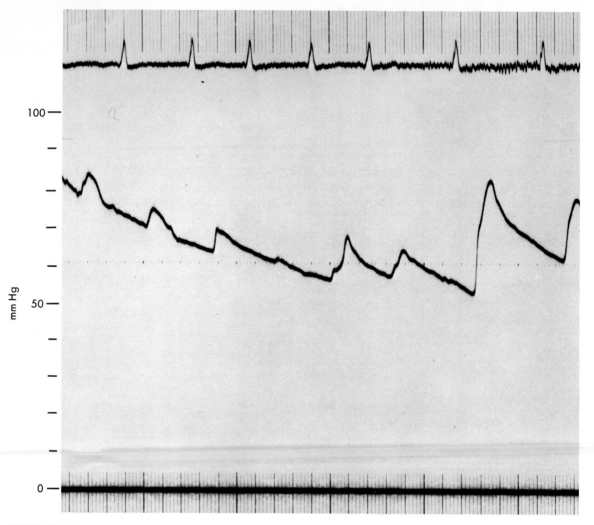

FIGURE 5-8

ANALYSIS

Rhythm: Atrial fibrillation

Pressure(s): (?) Possibly arterial

Waveform characteristics and measurements:

1. _____ ; _____ mm Hg
2. _____ ; _____ mm Hg
3. _____ ; _____ mm Hg
4. _____ ; _____ mm Hg
5. _____ ; _____ mm Hg
6. _____ ; _____ mm Hg
7. _____ ; _____ mm Hg

Suspected abnormality/diagnosis: Inaccurate arterial pressure

Comments: The stopcock from the patient to the transducer is only partially open resulting in an erroneous arterial pressure.

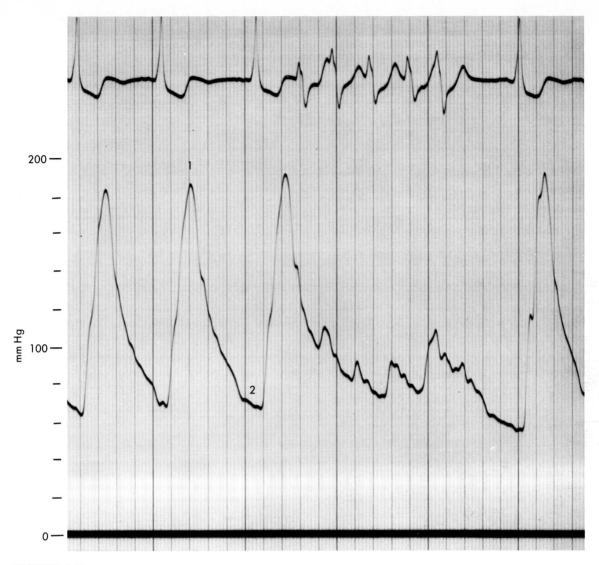

FIGURE 5-9

ANALYSIS

Rhythm: NSR with five-beat run of PVCs

Pressure(s): Radial artery

Waveform characteristics and measurements:

1.	Arterial systolic	;	180	mm Hg
2.	Arterial end-diastolic	;	60	mm Hg
3.		;		mm Hg
4.		;		mm Hg
5.		;		mm Hg
6.		;		mm Hg
7.		;		mm Hg

Suspected abnormality/diagnosis: Aortic regurgitation

Comments: Note the wide pulse pressure (120 mm Hg) and poorly defined or absent dicrotic notch, indicative of aortic regurgitation. Note also the devastating effects of a five-beat run of VT with a drop in arterial pressure to approximately 60 mm Hg, with minimal stroke volume.

103

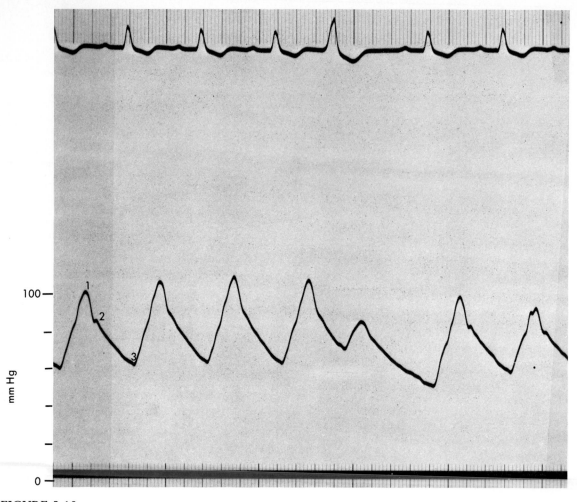

FIGURE 5-10

ANALYSIS

Rhythm: NSR with PVC

Pressure(s): Radial artery

Waveform characteristics and measurements:

1.	Arterial systolic	;	92	mm Hg
2.	Dicrotic notch	;		mm Hg
3.	Arterial end-diastolic	;	60	mm Hg
4.		;		mm Hg
5.		;		mm Hg
6.		;		mm Hg
7.		;		mm Hg

Suspected abnormality/diagnosis: Aortic stenosis

Comments: The slow upstroke of the arterial pulse in aortic stenosis is due to the resistance to ejection at the aortic valve. The poorly defined dicrotic notch is due to stiff movement and closure of the aortic valve leaflets. Additionally, the narrow pulse pressure indicates a small stroke volume. Note the even further decrease in pressure and stroke volume following a premature ventricular beat, which reduces the amount of time for LV filling.

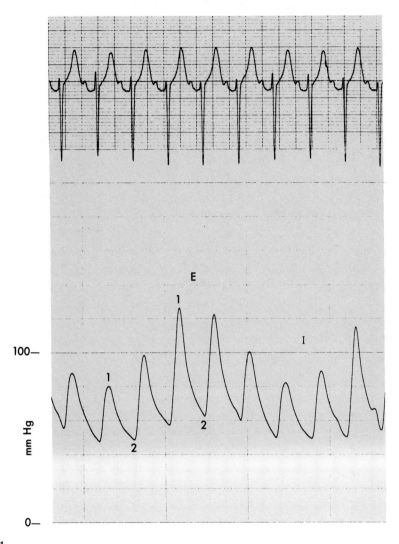

FIGURE 5-11

ANALYSIS

Rhythm: Sinus tachycardia

Pressure(s): Radial artery

Waveform characteristics and measurements:

1.	Systolic	;	80-125	mm Hg
2.	Diastolic	;	50-60	mm Hg
3.		;		mm Hg
4.		;		mm Hg
5.		;		mm Hg
6.		;		mm Hg
7.		;		mm Hg

Suspected abnormality/diagnosis: Cardiac tamponade

Comments: Note the exaggerated decline in the arterial systolic pressure during inspiration *(I)*. This is termed pulsus paradoxus and, classically, occurs in cardiac tamponade.

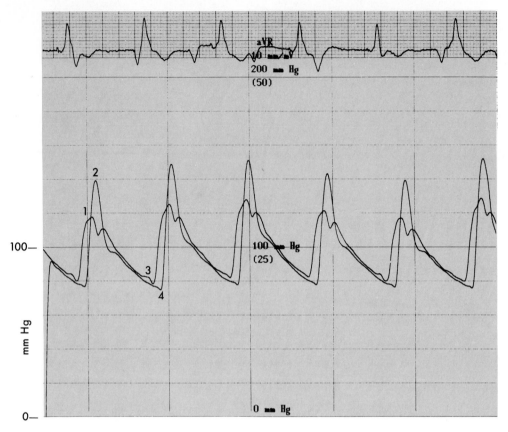

FIGURE 5-12

ANALYSIS

Rhythm: Complete heart block

Pressure(s): Ascending aortic and femoral artery

Waveform characteristics and measurements:

1.	Aortic systolic	;	120	mm Hg
2.	Femoral artery systolic	;	142	mm Hg
3.	Aortic diastolic	;	80	mm Hg
4.	Femoral artery diastolic	;	75	mm Hg
5.		;		mm Hg
6.		;		mm Hg
7.		;		mm Hg

Suspected abnormality/diagnosis: Normal arterial pressures

Comments: Simultaneous recording of the ascending aortic and femoral artery pressures reveals the normal discrepancy between central and peripheral arterial pressures as the pulse wave travels distally.

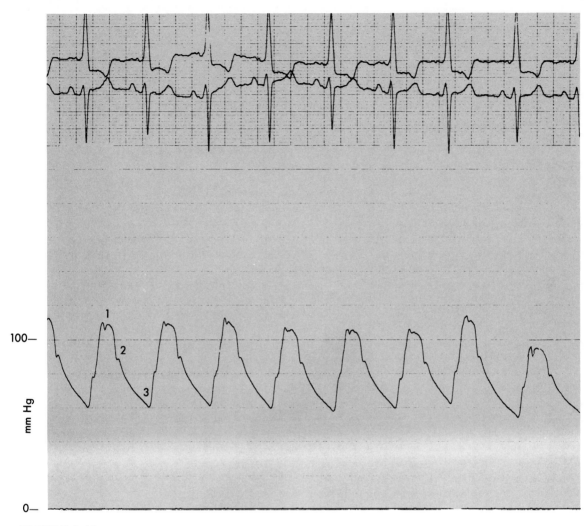

100—

mm Hg

0—

FIGURE 5-13

ANALYSIS

Rhythm: NSR

Pressure(s): Radial artery

Waveform characteristics and measurements:

1.	Systolic	;	110	mm Hg
2.	Dicrotic notch	;		mm Hg
3.	Diastolic	;	60	mm Hg
4.		;		mm Hg
5.		;		mm Hg
6.		;		mm Hg
7.		;		mm Hg

Suspected abnormality/diagnosis: Hypertrophic cardiomyopathy

Comments: The systolic pressure of this arterial waveform has a double-peak or bifid appearance, a feature commonly seen in patients with hypertrophic cardiomyopathy.

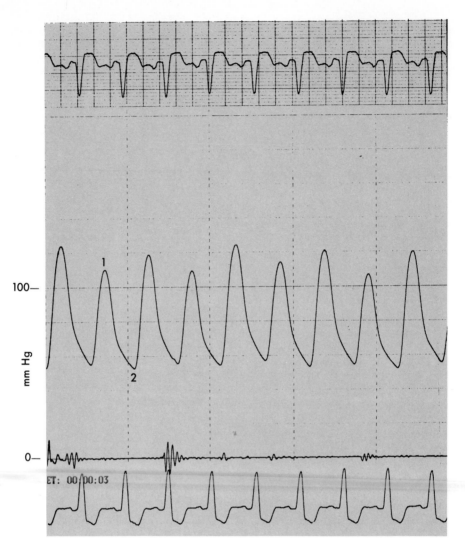

FIGURE 5-14

ANALYSIS

Rhythm: NSR

Pressure(s): Femoral artery

Waveform characteristics and measurements:

1.	Systolic	;	110-120	mm Hg
2.	Diastolic	;	55	mm Hg
3.		;		mm Hg
4.		;		mm Hg
5.		;		mm Hg
6.		;		mm Hg
7.		;		mm Hg

Suspected abnormality/diagnosis: LV failure

Comments: This arterial waveform has a regular, alternating change in the systolic pressure. This is termed pulsus alternans and commonly is associated with severe LV failure.

Chapter 6

Patient Profiles

Invasive hemodynamic monitoring is used in a variety of clinical situations. It can be helpful in the diagnosis of certain pathologic conditions, such as pulmonary embolus or ventricular septal defect (VSD). (With pulmonary embolus the PAedp is elevated, whereas the PAWm may be normal or low; with a VSD the oxygen saturation of a blood sample from the PA will be higher than an RA blood oxygen saturation.) Its major application, however, remains as a continuous assessment of the cardiovascular state of high-risk medical or surgical situations (myocardial infarction, openheart surgery, high-risk general surgery, ARDS, and burns). Hemodynamic data provide detailed, finely focused information that serves as an adjunct to the broader picture obtained through clinical assessment. Additionally, it offers a means of immediately evaluating the effectiveness or ineffectiveness of therapeutic interventions. Administration of certain pharmacologic agents can be carefully individualized and titrated according to the hemodynamic response.

This chapter presents multiple patient profiles to illustrate the varied situations in which invasive hemodynamic monitoring is employed and hemodynamic responses to certain therapeutic agents. Additionally, it provides the opportunity for furthering skills in waveform identification and interpretation.

Patient Profile 1

A 58-year-old woman was transferred via air evacuation from a community hospital where she had been admitted for chest pains accompanied by ST elevation in the inferior leads and initially treated with nitroglycerine (both sublingual and intravenous infusion), morphine, and heparin. Past medical history included prosthetic aortic and mitral valve replacements 3 years ago for valvular heart disease secondary to rheumatic fever. Postoperative complications included a possible myocardial infarction (MI) and cerebrovascular accident (CVA). The patient had been receiving Coumadin until it was discontinued because of gastrointestinal bleeding several months before admission.

On examination, the blood pressure was 102/72, heart rate was 100 beats/min, and respiratory rate as 12 breaths/min. Jugular venous pressure was approximately 10 to 11 cm with normal carotid upstrokes. Cardiac exam revealed a diffuse, somewhat lateral point of maximal impulse (PMI), a normal S_1 and S_2, and a grade 1/6 systolic ejection murmur heard at the lower left sternal border. The lungs were clear,and trace peripheral edema was evident with diminished peripheral pulses. The patient was oriented, although quite lethargic. Laboratory values were remarkable for a hemoglobin of 9.2 gm/dl and a partial thromboplastin time (PTT) of 39.4 seconds. Hemodynamic assessment via the PA catheter revealed a cardiac output of 2.9 L/min, with a cardiac index of 1.9 L/min/m^2 and an a-vO$_2$ difference of 5.6 vol%. In addition, the following hemodynamic pressures were obtained (Figures 6-1 to 6-4).

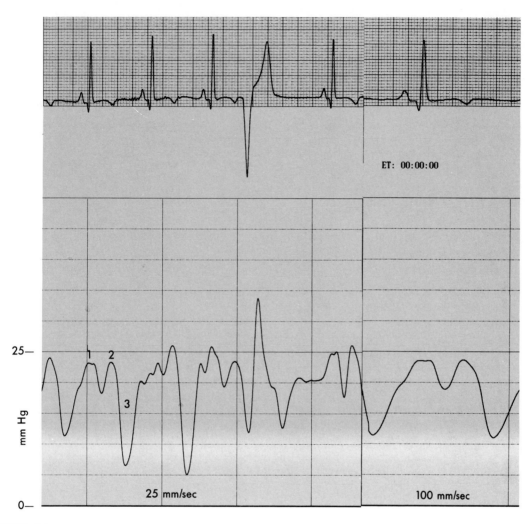

ET: 00:00:00

25—

mm Hg

0—

25 mm/sec   100 mm/sec

FIGURE 6-1

ANALYSIS

Rhythm: NSR with PVC

Pressure(s): RA

Waveform characteristics and measurements:

1.	*a* Wave	;	24	mm Hg
2.	*v* Wave	;	24	mm Hg
3.	*y* Descent	;		mm Hg
4.	Mean	;	19	mm Hg
5.		;		mm Hg
6.		;		mm Hg
7.		;		mm Hg

Suspected abnormality/diagnosis: RV failure secondary to RV infarction

Comments: Note the exaggerated *y* descent of this RA waveform. This constrictive pattern in the RA waveform is seen commonly in association with RV infarction. Note, also, the increased paper speed (100 mm/sec) for the last beat which aids in accurately identifying the *a* and *v* waves.

113

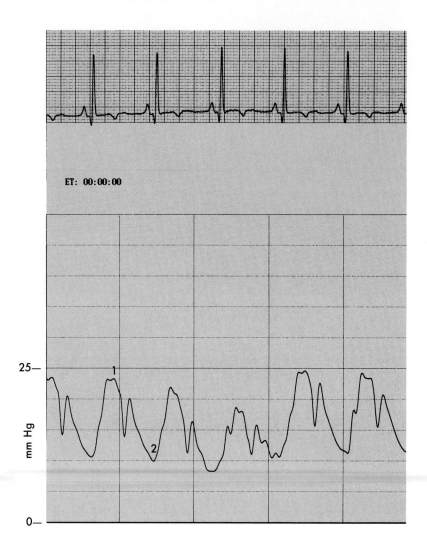

FIGURE 6-2

ANALYSIS

Rhythm: NSR

Pressure(s): PA

Waveform characteristics and measurements:

1.	Systolic	;	21	mm Hg
2.	End-diastolic	;	11	mm Hg
3.		;		mm Hg
4.		;		mm Hg
5.		;		mm Hg
6.		;		mm Hg
7.		;		mm Hg

Suspected abnormality/diagnosis: RV failure secondary to RV infarction

Comments: Although this PA pressure is normal in both contour and value, the small pulse pressure of 10 mm Hg suggests diminished stroke volume from the right ventricle as a result of RV infarction.

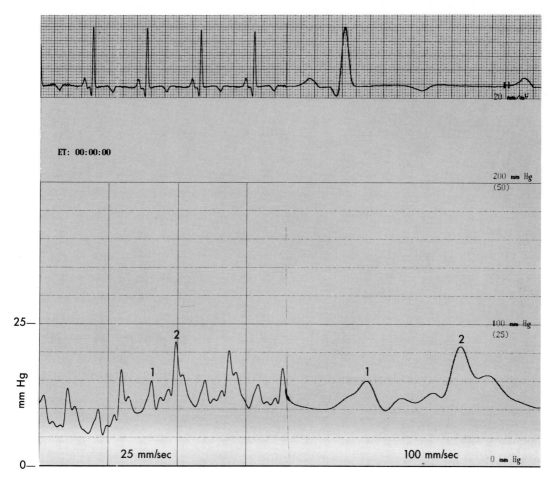

FIGURE 6-3

ANALYSIS

Rhythm: NSR

Pressure(s): PAW

Waveform characteristics and measurements:

1.	a Wave	;	13	mm Hg
2.	v Wave	;	17	mm Hg
3.	Mean	;	13	mm Hg
4.		;		mm Hg
5.		;		mm Hg
6.		;		mm Hg
7.		;		mm Hg

Suspected abnormality/diagnosis: RV failure secondary to RV infarction

Comments: This PAW pressure is basically normal indicating LV failure is not the cause of this patient's cardiac dysfunction. The v wave is slightly dominant with a slow y descent. These findings are consistent with a prosthetic mitral valve. The mean pressure of 13 mm Hg suggests that the administration of volume to increase preload and, thus, stroke volume, could be done quite safely.

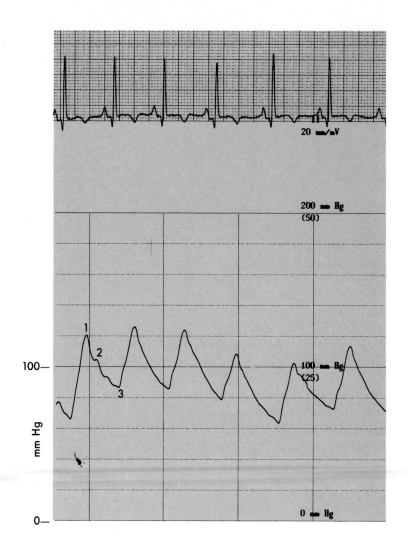

FIGURE 6-4

ANALYSIS

Rhythm: NSR

Pressure(s): Radial artery

Waveform characteristics and measurements:

1.	Systolic	;	115	mm Hg
2.	Dicrotic notch	;		mm Hg
3.	Diastolic	;	80	mm Hg
4.		;		mm Hg
5.		;		mm Hg
6.		;		mm Hg
7.		;		mm Hg

Suspected abnormality/diagnosis: RV failure secondary to RV infarction

Comments: Although this radial artery pressure appears to have a somewhat damped appearance with a slow upstroke and poorly defined dicrotic notch, this could be due to the function of the prosthetic aortic valve.

116

Patient Profile 2

A 69-year-old woman was admitted to the emergency room complaining of several hours of severe chest pressure without associated nausea, vomiting, shortness of breath, palpitations, or dizziness. Past medical history included an anterior subendocardial myocardial infarction (MI) 2 years previously. The patient was a smoker of 30 years and was being treated for chronic hypertension.

Blood pressure was 120/70, heart rate was 64 beats/min, and respiratory rate was 18 breaths/min. Scant bilateral basilar rales were heard; neck veins were flat; and an S_4 was detected with an otherwise normal cardiovascular examination. The admission ECG showed ST depression in the anterolateral leads. She was admitted to the coronary care unit (CCU) where routine MI management was carried out including oxygen, lidocaine infusion, heparin, and morphine. Serial enzymes at 36 hours postadmission showed a creatine phosphokinase (CPK) value of 430 with an MB of 25% and a lactate dehydrogenase (LDH) value of 291. The patient was stable for 2 days when she suddenly complained of recurrent chest pressure and severe dyspnea. Blood pressure was palpable at 80 mm Hg, heart rate was 106 beats/min, and respiratory rate was 28 breaths/min. She was cyanotic, cold and clammy, and slightly confused. Rales were present bilaterally to the apices. A left parasternal thrill and a grade 5/6 systolic murmur were heard. On 2 L O_2/min the arterial blood gas revealed a pO_2 of 32 mm Hg, a pCO_2 of 38 mm Hg and a pH of 7.46. The patient was intubated and given 100% O_2 initially. Dopamine infusion was begun at 10 mcg/kg/min. The ECG revealed prominent ST depression in leads V2-4. The chest x-ray revealed bilateral interstitial and alveolar infiltrates. A PA catheter was inserted and the hemodynamic data included a cardiac output of 2.6 L/min, with a cardiac index of 1.5 L/min/m^2 and an a-vO_2 difference of 8.6 vol% in addition to the following hemodynamic pressures (Figures 6-5 to 6-8).

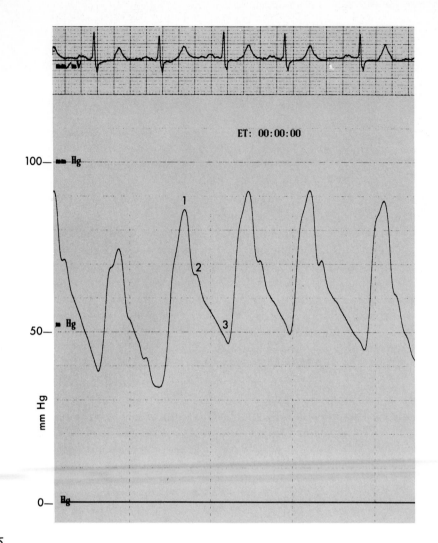

ET: 00:00:00

100— mm Hg

mm Hg

50— mm Hg

0— Hg

FIGURE 6-5

ANALYSIS

Rhythm: NSR

Pressure(s): Radial artery

Waveform characteristics and measurements:

1.	Systolic	;	88	mm Hg
2.	Dicrotic notch	;		mm Hg
3.	Diastolic	;	45	mm Hg
4.		;		mm Hg
5.		;		mm Hg
6.		;		mm Hg
7.		;		mm Hg

Suspected abnormality/diagnosis: Hypotension

Comments: Although this radial artery pressure is normal in contour, the pressure is very low. The calculated coronary perfusion pressure (CPP) in this patient is approximately 10 mm Hg (arterial diastolic - RAm [35 mm Hg]), which is inadequate to maintain coronary perfusion.

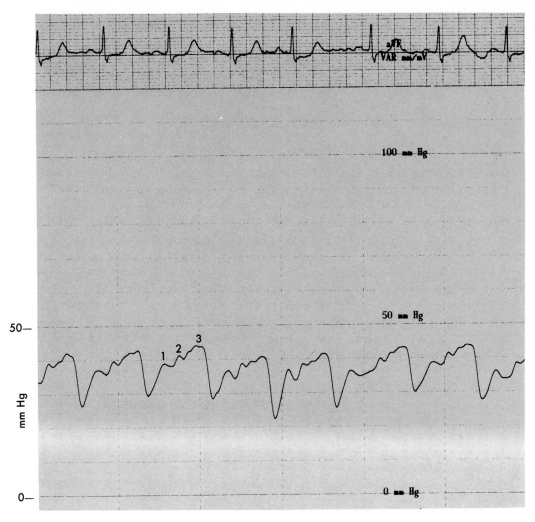

FIGURE 6-6

ANALYSIS

Rhythm: NSR

Pressure(s): RA

Waveform characteristics and measurements:

1.	*a* Wave	;	35	mm Hg
2.	*c* Wave	;		mm Hg
3.	*v* Wave	;	42	mm Hg
4.	Mean	;	35	mm Hg
5.		;		mm Hg
6.		;		mm Hg
7.		;		mm Hg

Suspected abnormality/diagnosis: Right heart failure

Comments: This RA pressure is markedly elevated suggesting severe right heart failure with volume overload.

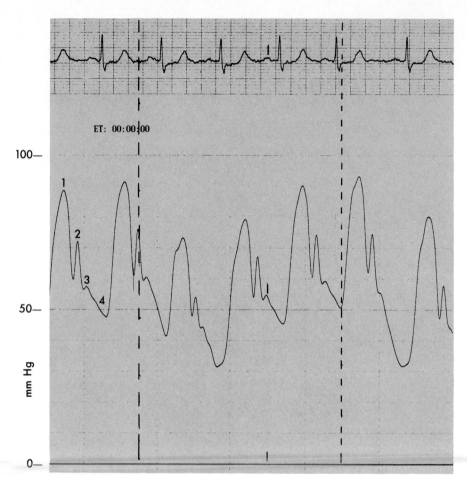

ET: 00:00:00

FIGURE 6-7

ANALYSIS

Rhythm: NSR
Pressure(s): PA
Waveform characteristics and measurements:

1.	Systolic	;	84	mm Hg
2.	Retrograde *v* wave	;	60	mm Hg
3.	Dicrotic notch	;		mm Hg
4.	Diastolic	;	42	mm Hg
5.		;		mm Hg
6.		;		mm Hg
7.		;		mm Hg

Suspected abnormality/diagnosis: Pulmonary hypertension secondary to severe LV failure and mitral regurgitation

Comments: This markedly elevated PA pressure is due to LV failure with severe mitral regurgitation. The first dotted line drawn after the T wave of the ECG reveals the presence of a superimposed retrograde *v* wave from the left atrium. The second dotted line immediately following the QRS complex indicates the beginning of systole and the upstroke of the PA waveform.

120

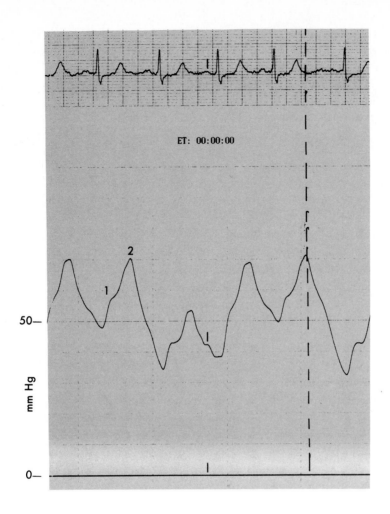

ET: 00:00:00

FIGURE 6-8

ANALYSIS

Rhythm: NSR

Pressure(s): PAW

Waveform characteristics and measurements:

1.	*a* Wave	; 50	mm Hg
2.	*v* Wave	; 65	mm Hg
3.		;	mm Hg
4.		;	mm Hg
5.		;	mm Hg
6.		;	mm Hg
7.		;	mm Hg

Suspected abnormality/diagnosis: LV failure with severe mitral regurgitation

Comments: The early appearance of this markedly elevated *v* wave almost obscures the *a* wave, thus altering the configuration of this PAW pressure. However, relating its timing to the ECG post T-wave period aids in accurate identification of this elevated *v* wave due to severe mitral regurgitation.

Patient Profile 3

An 18-year-old man with a history of cardiomyopathy of unknown etiology was admitted to the CCU with hypotension and symptoms of both right- and left-sided heart failure.

On examination, the patient was dyspneic with a respiratory rate of 24 breaths/min. Cardiovascular exam revealed jugular venous distention of approximately 12 cm with an RV lift and laterally displaced PMI. Heart sounds S_1 and S_2 were normal, and both an S_3 and S_4 were present. A grade 4/6 systolic ejection murmur was heard at the left sternal border. Bilateral rales were present in the lower third of the lungs. A PA and an arterial catheter were inserted and revealed a cardiac index of 1.2 L/min/m^2 in addition to the following hemodynamic pressure tracings (Figures 6-9 to 6-13).

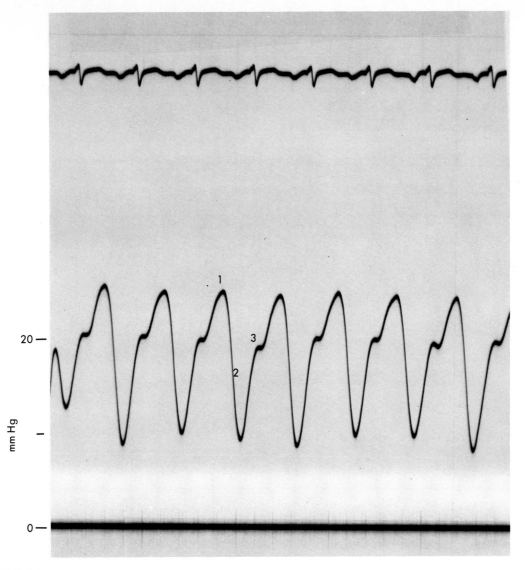

FIGURE 6-9

ANALYSIS

Rhythm: Sinus tachycardia

Pressure(s): RA

Waveform characteristics and measurements:

1.	*v* Wave	;	25	mm Hg
2.	*y* Descent	;		mm Hg
3.	*a* Wave	;	20	mm Hg
4.		;		mm Hg
5.		;		mm Hg
6.		;		mm Hg
7.		;		mm Hg

Suspected abnormality/diagnosis: RV failure with mild tricuspid regurgitation

Comments: The RA *v* wave is elevated and dominant with a rapid *y* descent, suggesting tricuspid regurgitation, probably functional and secondary to RV dilatation and failure. The elevated *a* wave indicates increased resistance to ventricular filling due to RV failure.

123

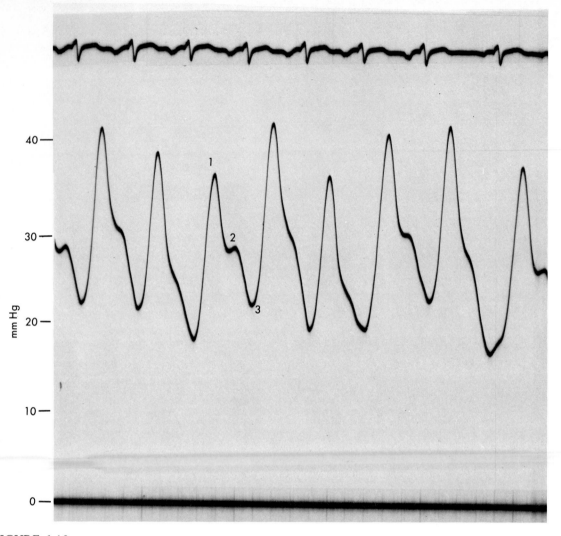

FIGURE 6-10

ANALYSIS

Rhythm: NSR

Pressure(s): PA

Waveform characteristics and measurements:

1.	PA systolic	;	40	mm Hg
2.	Dicrotic notch	;		mm Hg
3.	PA end-diastolic	;	23	mm Hg
4.		;		mm Hg
5.		;		mm Hg
6.		;		mm Hg
7.		;		mm Hg

Suspected abnormality/diagnosis: Pulmonary hypertension secondary to LV failure

Comments: This elevated PA pressure suggests the presence of LV as well as RV failure. Note the respiratory variation in the PA waveform with a rather rapid respiratory rate.

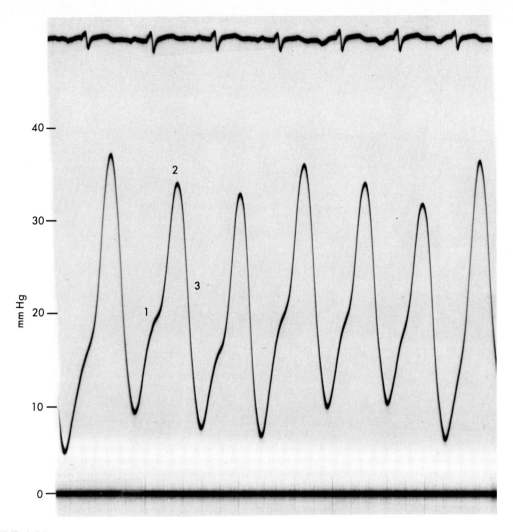

FIGURE 6-11

ANALYSIS

Rhythm: NSR

Pressure(s): PAW

Waveform characteristics and measurements:

1.	*a* Wave	;	20	mm Hg
2.	*v* Wave	;	37	mm Hg
3.	*y* Descent	;		mm Hg
4.		;		mm Hg
5.		;		mm Hg
6.		;		mm Hg
7.		;		mm Hg

Suspected abnormality/diagnosis: LV failure and mitral regurgitation secondary to papillary muscle dysfunction

Comments: The early, dominant, and elevated PAW *v* wave virtually obscures the PAW *a* wave. The rapid *y* descent following the large *v* wave is characteristic of mitral regurgitation and is due to the early, facile emptying of the left atrium. Note the correlation of the PAW *a* wave to the PAedp in Figure 6-10.

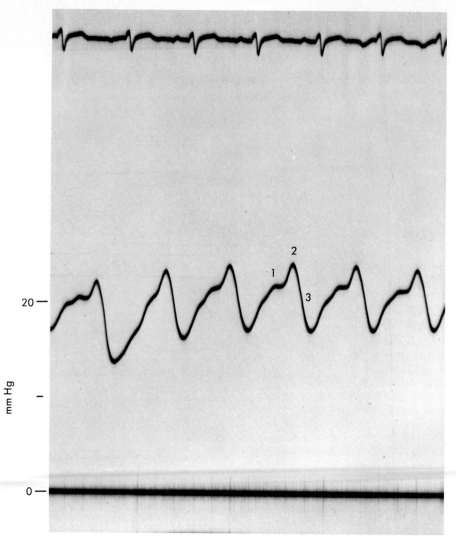

FIGURE 6-12

ANALYSIS

Rhythm: NSR

Pressure(s): PAW

Waveform characteristics and measurements:

1.	*a* Wave	;	21	mm Hg
2.	*v* Wave	;	25	mm Hg
3.	*y* Descent	;		mm Hg
4.		;		mm Hg
5.		;		mm Hg
6.		;		mm Hg
7.		;		mm Hg

Suspected abnormality/diagnosis: LV failure with mild to moderate mitral regurgitation

Comments: This patient was treated with nitroprusside in an attempt to increase forward flow and reduce the regurgitant volume by reducing afterload. Compare this PAW pressure to the previous PAW pressure tracing (Figure 6-11) and note the marked decrease in the *v* wave from 35 to 26 mm Hg.

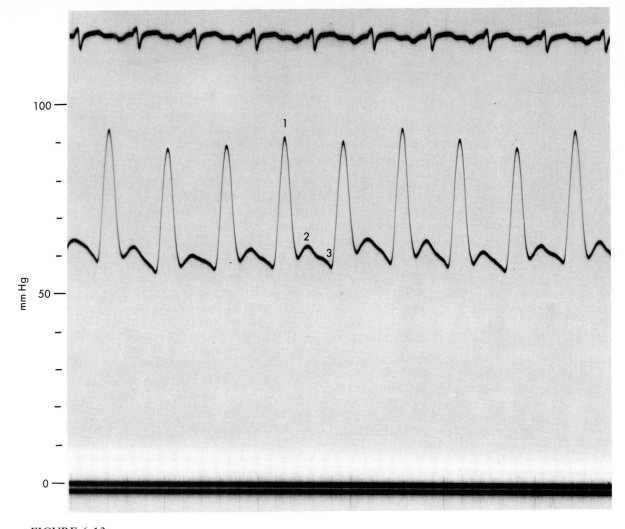

FIGURE 6-13

ANALYSIS

Rhythm: Sinus tachycardia

Pressure(s): Radial artery

Waveform characteristics and measurements:

1.	Peak systolic	;	92	mm Hg
2.	Dicrotic notch	;		mm Hg
3.	End-diastolic	;	55	mm Hg
4.		;		mm Hg
5.		;		mm Hg
6.		;		mm Hg
7.		;		mm Hg

Suspected abnormality/diagnosis: Hypotension with nitroprusside therapy

Comments: The contour of this arterial pressure is somewhat unusual as a result of the tachycardia, which shortens the duration of diastolic runoff, and the induced vasodilatation, which increases stroke volume (by decreasing resistance) and facilitates rapid runoff peripherally.

Patient Profile 4

A 38-year-old woman with a history of pulmonary hypertension and severe bradycardia with syncope treated with a permanent pacemaker was admitted for evaluation of pacemaker function as well as symptoms of congestive heart failure with marked dyspnea on exertion and lower extremity edema. The patient had undergone several pacemaker replacements over the last 10 years. At the time of the first replacement, the original pacemaker lead could not be removed. On the subsequent replacement one end of this lead was noted to be floating in the superior vena cava (SVC), but still could not be removed.

On examination, jugular venous distention was present to above the angle of the jaw. Cardiovascular examination revealed a laterally displaced PMI with a prominent RV heave. Heart sounds included a normal S_1 and S_2 with a loud right-sided S_3, and grade 3/6 decrescendo murmur and a grade 2/6 systolic ejection murmur at the left upper–sternal border. Abdominal examination revealed an enlarged and tender liver. Moderate (2+) peripheral edema was present with diminished pulsations.

A PA catheter was inserted to determine the degree of right heart failure. The patient's thermodilution cardiac output was 1.6 L/min, with a cardiac index of 1.1 L/min/m^2, and her a-vO$_2$ difference was 11.1 vol%. The following hemodynamic pressures were obtained (Figures 6-14 to 6-17).

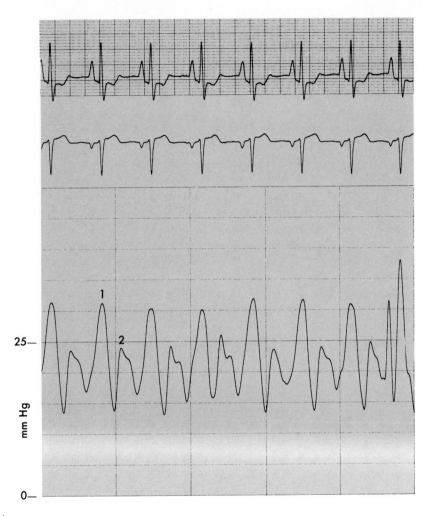

FIGURE 6-14

ANALYSIS

Rhythm: NSR
Pressure(s): RA
Waveform characteristics and measurements:

1.	*a* Wave	;	31	mm Hg
2.	*v* Wave	;	23	mm Hg
3.	Mean	;	23	mm Hg
4.		;		mm Hg
5.		;		mm Hg
6.		;		mm Hg
7.		;		mm Hg

Suspected abnormality/diagnosis: Right heart failure

Comments: The dominant, elevated *a* wave of 31 mm Hg indicates severe right heart failure.

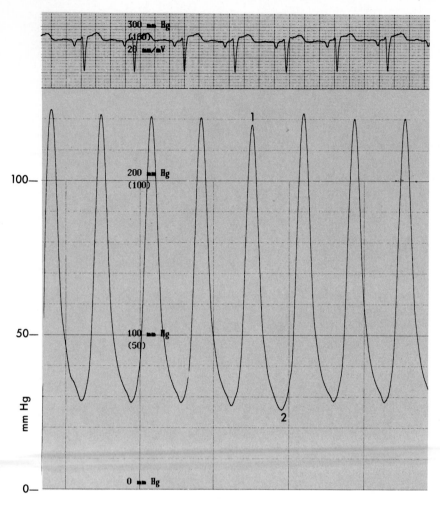

FIGURE 6-15

ANALYSIS

Rhythm: NSR

Pressure(s): PA

Waveform characteristics and measurements:

1.	Systolic	; 120	mm Hg
2.	Diastolic	; 28	mm Hg
3.		;	mm Hg
4.		;	mm Hg
5.		;	mm Hg
6.		;	mm Hg
7.		;	mm Hg

Suspected abnormality/diagnosis: Severe pulmonary hypertension with pulmonic insufficiency

Comments: This markedly elevated PA pressure bears the classic features of valvular regurgitation with a wide pulse pressure (92 mm Hg) and absent dicrotic notch. The severe pulmonary hypertension is due to chronic multiple pulmonary emboli from the pacemaker wire. The pulmonic regurgitation is a result of coiling of the free pacemaker wire through the pulmonic valve.

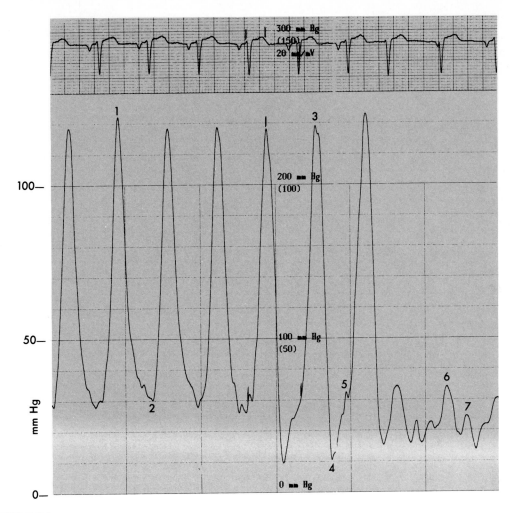

FIGURE 6-16

ANALYSIS

Rhythm: NSR

Pressure(s): PA/RV/RA

Waveform characteristics and measurements:

1.	PA systolic	;	120	mm Hg
2.	PA diastolic	;	30	mm Hg
3.	RV systolic	;	120	mm Hg
4.	RV diastolic	;	10	mm Hg
5.	RV end-diastolic	;	33	mm Hg
6.	RA *a* wave	;	34	mm Hg
7.	RA *v* wave	;	24	mm Hg

Suspected abnormality/diagnosis: Severe pulmonary hypertension with pulmonic insufficiency

Comments: Because of the severe pulmonic regurgitation the PA catheter migrates back into the RV and on into the RA. Maintaining placement of the catheter tip in the PA is likely not possible in this situation.

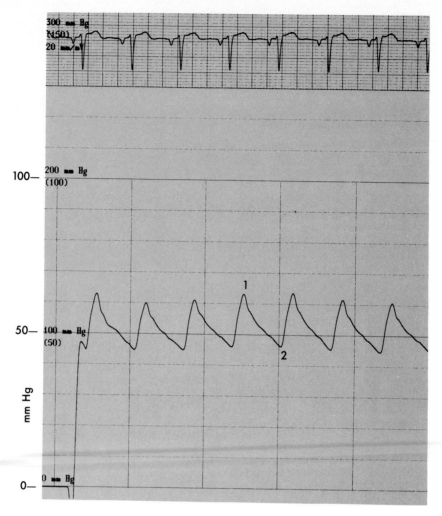

FIGURE 6-17

ANALYSIS

Rhythm: NSR

Pressure(s): Radial artery

Waveform characteristics and measurements:

1.	Systolic	;	20	mm Hg
2.	Diastolic	;	90	mm Hg
3.	Mean	;	100	mm Hg
4.		;		mm Hg
5.		;		mm Hg
6.		;		mm Hg
7.		;		mm Hg

Suspected abnormality/diagnosis: Pulmonary hypertension with pulmonic insufficiency

Comments: This moderately reduced arterial pressure reflects the low stroke volume as a result of reduced filling of the left heart because of the severe pulmonic insufficiency.

132

Patient Profile 5

A 27-year-old woman was admitted to the CCU with marked hypotension and increasing symptoms of both right- and left-sided heart failure, including dyspnea, ascites, and cyanosis. Past medical history included a myomectomy and prosthetic mitral valve replacement 6 years previously for idiopathic hypertrophic subaortic stenosis (IHSS). A temporary demand pacemaker was inserted, and hemodynamic instrumentation was initiated. The patient's cardiac index was 1.2 L/min/m^2, and the following hemodynamic pressures were obtained (Figures 6-18 to 6-23).

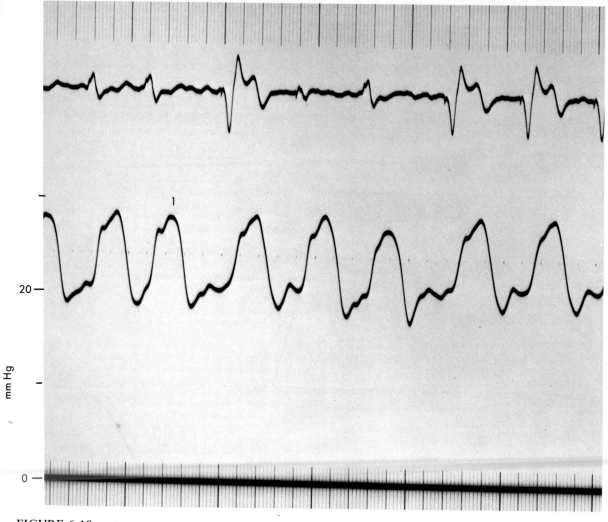

FIGURE 6-18

ANALYSIS

Rhythm: Atrial fibrillation with temporary demand pacemaker at 70 BPM

Pressure(s): RA

Waveform characteristics and measurements:

1.	v Wave	; 30 mm Hg
2.		; mm Hg
3.		; mm Hg
4.		; mm Hg
5.		; mm Hg
6.		; mm Hg
7.		; mm Hg

Suspected abnormality/diagnosis: RV failure with severe tricuspid regurgitation

Comments: The presence of atrial fibrillation accounts for the lack of an *a* wave in this RA pressure waveform. The elevated *v* wave of 30 mm Hg is due to regurgitation of blood into the RA during RV systole. This is probably functional tricuspid regurgitation secondary to a dilated right ventricle. Although there is no *a* wave present, the fact that the pressure never falls below 20 mm Hg indicates RV failure.

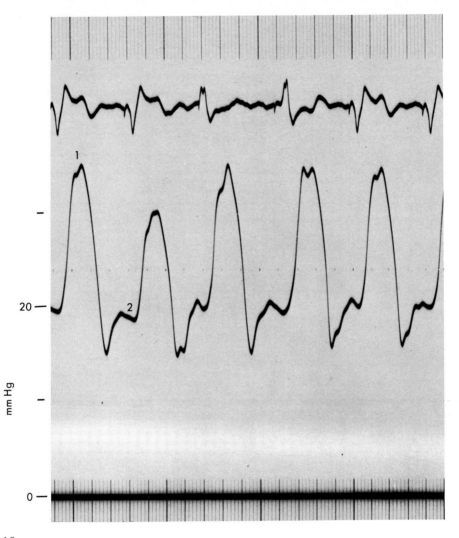

FIGURE 6-19

ANALYSIS

Rhythm: Atrial fibrillation with temporary demand pacemaker at 70 BPM

Pressure(s): RV

Waveform characteristics and measurements:

1.	RV systolic	;	35	mm Hg
2.	RV end-diastolic	;	20	mm Hg
3.		;		mm Hg
4.		;		mm Hg
5.		;		mm Hg
6.		;		mm Hg
7.		;		mm Hg

Suspected abnormality/diagnosis: RV failure

Comments: The RV systolic pressure is only mildly elevated (35 mm Hg), but the RV end-diastolic pressure of 20 mm Hg is indicative of severe RV failure.

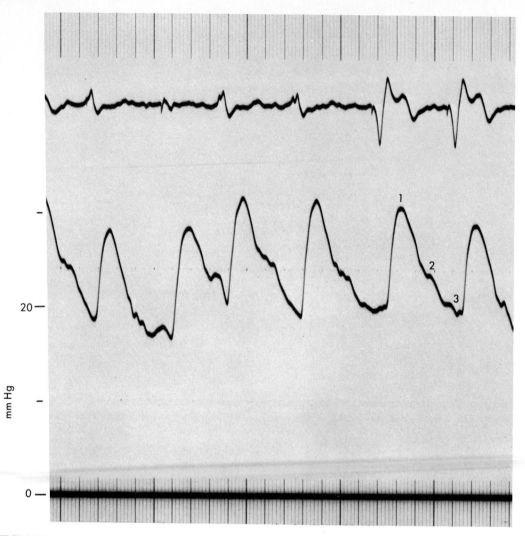

FIGURE 6-20

ANALYSIS

Rhythm: Atrial fibrillation with temporary demand pacemaker at 70 BPM

Pressure(s): PA

Waveform characteristics and measurements:

1.	PA systolic	; 32	mm Hg
2.	Dicrotic notch	;	mm Hg
3.	PA end-diastolic	; 20	mm Hg
4.		;	mm Hg
5.		;	mm Hg
6.		;	mm Hg
7.		;	mm Hg

Suspected abnormality/diagnosis: LV failure

Comments: The PA systolic pressure is only mildly elevated, possibly due to diminished forward blood flow from the RV. The end-diastolic pressure of 20 mm Hg is moderately elevated, indicating mild LV failure in addition to RV failure.

136

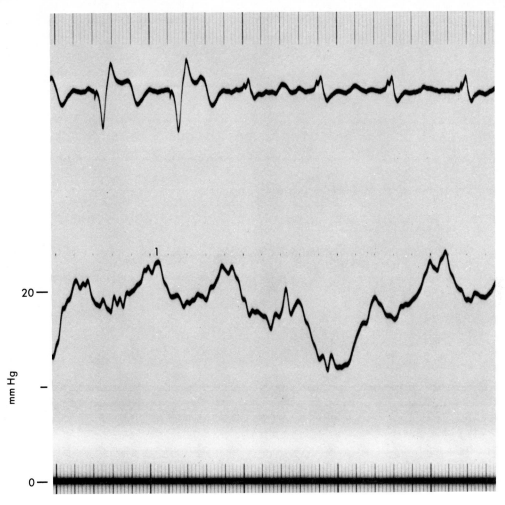

FIGURE 6-21

ANALYSIS

Rhythm: Atrial fibrillation with temporary demand pacemaker at 70 BPM
Pressure(s): PAW
Waveform characteristics and measurements:

1.	v Wave	; 22	mm Hg
2.	Mean	; 20	mm Hg
3.		;	mm Hg
4.		;	mm Hg
5.		;	mm Hg
6.		;	mm Hg
7.		;	mm Hg

Suspected abnormality/diagnosis: LV failure

Comments: The *a* wave is absent in this PAW pressure waveform due to atrial fibrillation. The elevated mean pressure of 20 mm Hg suggests mild LV failure.

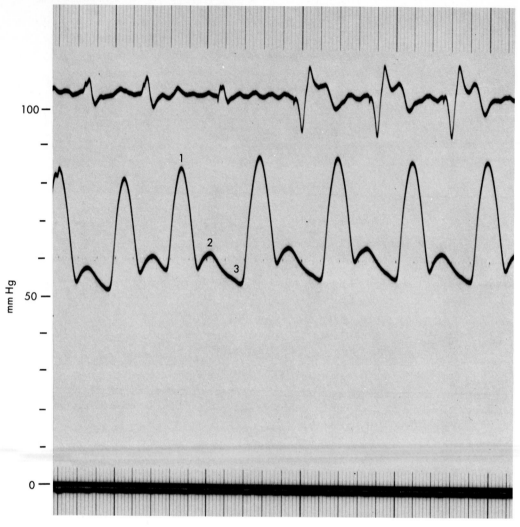

FIGURE 6-22

ANALYSIS

Rhythm: Atrial fibrillation/atrial flutter with demand pacemaker at 70 BPM

Pressure(s): Radial artery

Waveform characteristics and measurements:

1.	Arterial systolic	;	84	mm Hg
2.	Dicrotic notch	;		mm Hg
3.	Arterial end-diastolic	;	57	mm Hg
4.		;		mm Hg
5.		;		mm Hg
6.		;		mm Hg
7.		;		mm Hg

Suspected abnormality/diagnosis: Hypotension

Comments: This low arterial pressure with narrow pulse pressure (27 mm Hg) is due to a small stroke volume secondary to bilateral ventricular failure.

138

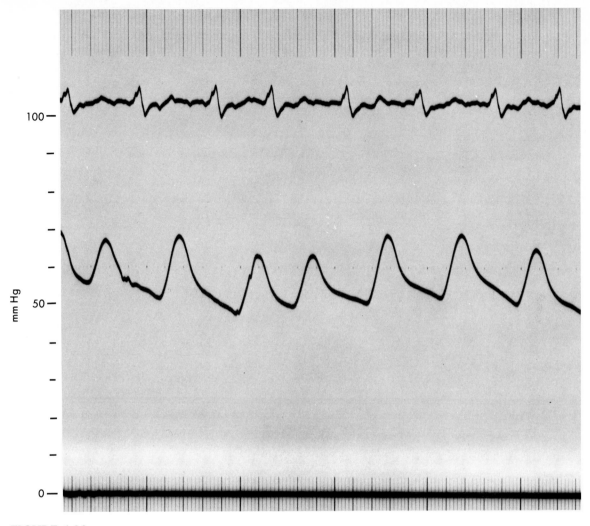

FIGURE 6-23

ANALYSIS

Rhythm: Atrial fibrillation

Pressure(s): Radial artery

Waveform characteristics and measurements:

1.	Arterial systolic	;	68	mm Hg
2.	Arterial end-diastolic	;	52	mm Hg
3.		;		mm Hg
4.		;		mm Hg
5.		;		mm Hg
6.		;		mm Hg
7.		;		mm Hg

Suspected abnormality/diagnosis: Damped arterial pressure

Comments: Comparison of this pressure with the arterial pressure waveform in Figure 6-22 shows a pressure of much lower value with a narrower pulse pressure. Additionally, the contour has a rounded appearance, a slow upstroke, and poorly defined dicrotic notch. This could be due to a clot at the tip of the catheter or lodging of the catheter tip against the wall of the artery. Catheter manipulation or aspiration and flushing may be required to improve this pressure waveform.

Patient Profile 6

A 41-year-old woman with the confirmed diagnosis of dilated cardiomyopathy and progressive biventricular heart failure was admitted for evaluation for possible cardiac transplantation. The patient had previously undergone both a mitral commissurotomy and prosthetic mitral valve replacement.

The jugular venous pressure was elevated to the jaw angle. Cardiovascular exam revealed a normal S_1, a loud pulmonic component of S_2, and an S_3. A grade 2/6 holosystolic murmur was heard at the apex with radiation to the axilla. Auscultation of the lungs revealed dullness at both bases. Marked ascites and 2+ pitting edema of the lower extremities were also present. Hemodynamic instrumentation was performed to assess the patient's response to vasodilator therapy. Hemodynamic data obtained were a cardiac index of 2.2 L/min/m^2 and the following pressure tracings (Figures 6-24 to 6-29).

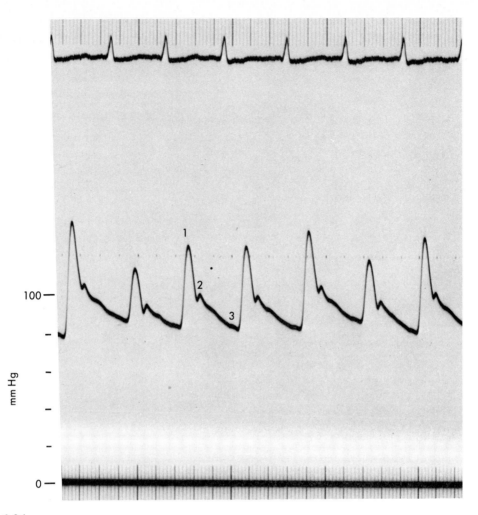

FIGURE 6-24

ANALYSIS

Rhythm: Atrial fibrillation

Pressure(s): Radial artery

Waveform characteristics and measurements:

1.	Arterial systolic	;	120	mm Hg
2.	Dicrotic notch	;		mm Hg
3.	Arterial diastolic	;	80	mm Hg
4.		;		mm Hg
5.		;		mm Hg
6.		;		mm Hg
7.		;		mm Hg

Suspected abnormality/diagnosis: Normal arterial pressure

Comments: Note the beat-to-beat variation in arterial pressure, reflecting changes in stroke volume, as a result of changes in filling time of the LV. The shorter the RR interval, the shorter the diastolic filling period and hence the lesser stroke volume. Compensatory vasoconstriction, which increases afterload, is responsible for maintaining this patient's blood pressure within normal levels.

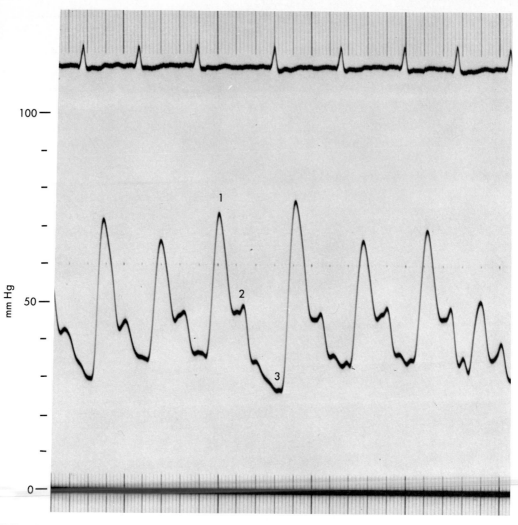

FIGURE 6-25

ANALYSIS

Rhythm: Atrial fibrillation

Pressure(s): PA

Waveform characteristics and measurements:

1.	PA systolic	;	66	mm Hg
2.	Dicrotic notch with superimposed v wave	;		mm Hg
3.	PA end-diastolic	;	30	mm Hg
4.		;		mm Hg
5.		;		mm Hg
6.		;		mm Hg
7.		;		mm Hg

Suspected abnormality/diagnosis: Pulmonary hypertension secondary to LV failure and mitral regurgitation

Comments: Note the extra notch on the dicrotic notch of this PA pressure. This represents retrograde transmission of an elevated v wave from the LA pressure due to mitral regurgitation. There is a more pronounced phase delay of this systolic event due to the retrograde transmission of the pressure. The elevated PAedp of 30 mm Hg indicates LV failure.

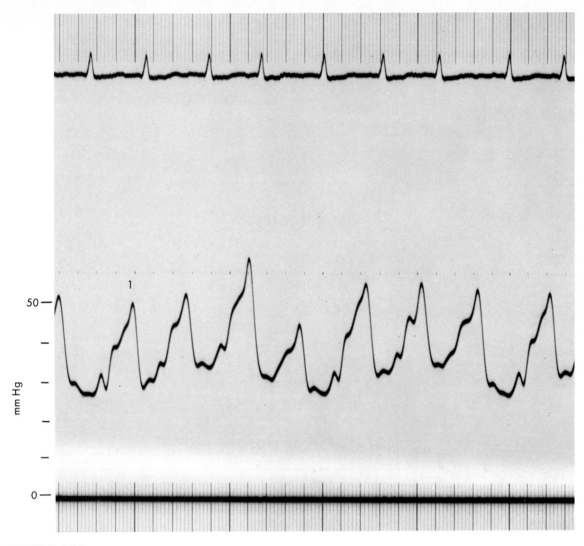

FIGURE 6-26

ANALYSIS

Rhythm: Atrial fibrillation

Pressure(s): PAW

Waveform characteristics and measurements:

1.	*v* Wave	;	50	mm Hg
2.		;		mm Hg
3.		;		mm Hg
4.		;		mm Hg
5.		;		mm Hg
6.		;		mm Hg
7.		;		mm Hg

Suspected abnormality/diagnosis: LV failure with mitral regurgitation

Comments: The loss of electrical atrial depolarization in atrial fibrillation results in a loss of mechanical atrial systole, and therefore no *a* waves are evident in this PAW pressure waveform. The numerous small waves preceding the *v* waves are probably fibrillatory waves. The elevated *v* wave of 50 mm Hg is due to mitral regurgitation, probably functional in nature. Note the similarity in the height of the *v* wave (approximately 50 mm Hg) and the superimposed *v* wave on the preceding PA pressure (Figure 6-25).

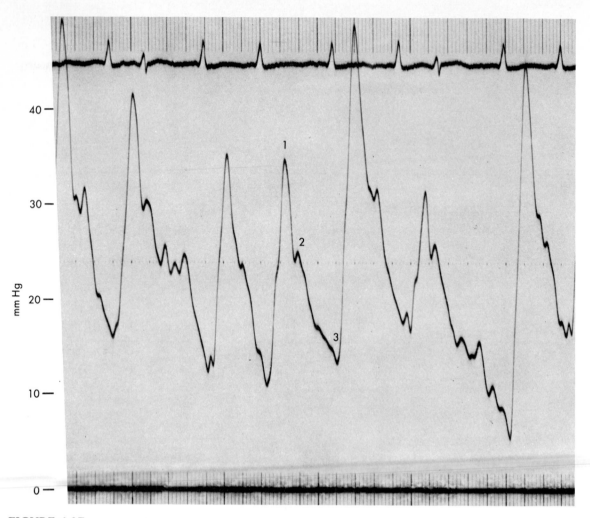

FIGURE 6-27

ANALYSIS

Rhythm: Atrial fibrillation

Pressure(s): PA

Waveform characteristics and measurements:

1.	PA systolic	;	40	mm Hg
2.	Dicrotic notch	;		mm Hg
3.	PA end-diastolic	;	15	mm Hg
4.		;		mm Hg
5.		;		mm Hg
6.		;		mm Hg
7.		;		mm Hg

Suspected abnormality/diagnosis: Mild pulmonary hypertension during afterload reduction

Comments: This PA pressure tracing is on a scale different from that of the PA pressure tracing in Figure 6-25, thus altering the overall appearance. The values of this PA pressure are lower, however, because of nitroprusside administration. The PAedp is now markedly reduced (from 30 to 15 mm Hg), indicating a decrease in LV preload due to enhanced forward output and venous pooling as a result of arterial and venous vasodilatation.

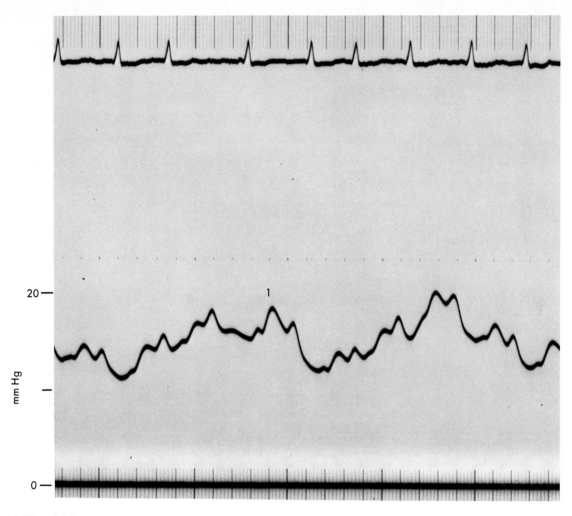

FIGURE 6-28

ANALYSIS

Rhythm: Atrial fibrillation

Pressure(s): PAW

Waveform characteristics and measurements:

1.	v Wave	; 18	mm Hg
2.	Mean	; 16	mm Hg
3.		;	mm Hg
4.		;	mm Hg
5.		;	mm Hg
6.		;	mm Hg
7.		;	mm Hg

Suspected abnormality/diagnosis: Improved PAW pressure during afterload reduction

Comments: This PAW pressure tracing is also recorded on a scale different from that of the previous PAW pressure (Figure 6-26). The v wave, however, is markedly reduced (from 47 to 18 mm Hg) because of nitroprusside therapy. This is due to afterload reduction, which has facilitated and enhanced forward blood flow and reduced retrograde blood flow into the left atrium. The mean pressure of 16 mm Hg indicates only mild congestive heart failure.

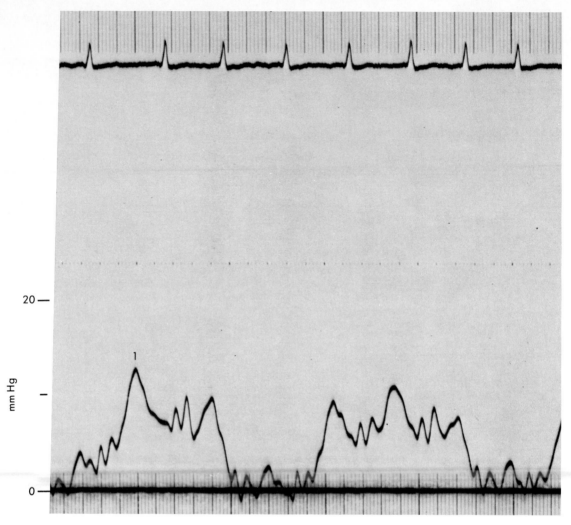

FIGURE 6-29

ANALYSIS

Rhythm: Atrial fibrillation

Pressure(s): PAW

Waveform characteristics and measurements:

1.	v Wave	;	8	mm Hg
2.	Mean	;	7	mm Hg
3.		;		mm Hg
4.		;		mm Hg
5.		;		mm Hg
6.		;		mm Hg
7.		;		mm Hg

Suspected abnormality/diagnosis: Relative hypovolemia secondary to afterload reduction

Comments: The further decrease in PAW pressure with continued nitroprusside administration may reflect a state of relative hypovolemia secondary to venodilatation and venous pooling. If there are concomitant signs of hypoperfusion, this low PAW pressure of 7 mm Hg might indicate the need for volume administration to maintain optimal preload levels.

Patient Profile 7

A 58-year-old man was admitted to the emergency room with a history of 2 hours of substernal chest pain and severe dyspnea. The patient had an inferior myocardial infarction (MI) 13 years ago and had a coronary artery bypass graft to his right coronary artery (RCA) and left anterior descending artery (LAD) 3 years ago. Since then, the patient has had occasional stable angina. The patient also has a history of hypertension as well as mitral regurgitation.

On examination, the patient was dyspneic with a respiratory rate of 22 breaths/min, a heart rate of 96 beats/min, and blood pressure of 130/70. Cardiovascular (CV) exam revealed 10 to 12 cm jugular venous distention with normal carotid upstrokes. The PMI was laterally displaced in the anterior axillary line. Heart sounds revealed a normal S_1, a soft S_2, an S_3, and possibly an S_4 with a grade 4/6 systolic ejection murmur. Bilateral basilar rales were present in the lower third of the lungs.

The patient was admitted to the CCU where an MI was ruled out by ECG and enzymes. A PA catheter was inserted to judiciously diurese the patient without jeopardizing LV function and cardiac output. Treatment of his congestive heart failure (CHF) consisted of nasal O_2 at 3 L/min and gentle diuresis with Lasix.

The hemodynamic data over the next few days are represented in the following hemodynamic pressures (Figures 6-30 to 6-31).

The patient remained stable until hospital day 3 when he suddenly became extremely dyspneic and agitated without complaints of chest pain. Hemodynamic data revealed a cardiac output of 2.31 L/min, with a cardiac index of 1.31 L/min/m^2, an a-vO_2 difference of 6.8 vol%, and the following hemodynamic pressures (Figures 6-32 to 6-33).

The patient was given a total of 50 mg Lasix intravenously over 30 mins and a nitroglycerine infusion was initiated at 10 mcg/min. Nasal O_2 was increased to 5 L/min. The hemodynamic data in Figure 6-34 were obtained approximately 1 hour later.

Nitroglycerine was subsequently decreased and eventually discontinued. An echocardiogram revealed severe ventricular dyskinesis with a severely dilated left ventricle and an ejection fraction of 17%.

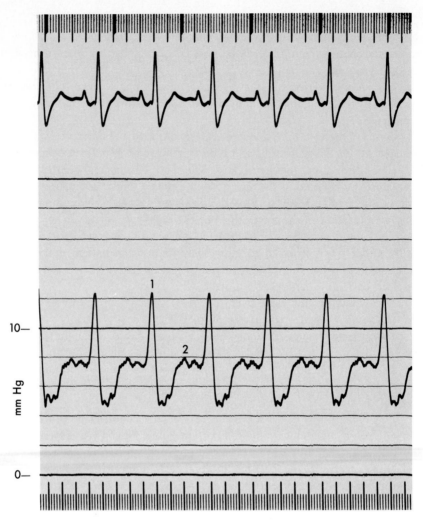

FIGURE 6-30

ANALYSIS

Rhythm: NSR

Pressure(s): RA

Waveform characteristics and measurements:

1.	*a* Wave	;	12	mm Hg
2.	*v* Wave	;	8	mm Hg
3.		;		mm Hg
4.		;		mm Hg
5.		;		mm Hg
6.		;		mm Hg
7.		;		mm Hg

Suspected abnormality/diagnosis: LV failure with mitral regurgitation

Comments: This RA waveform reveals a dominant and somewhat elevated *a* wave indicating mild RV failure secondary to longstanding LV failure and mitral regurgitation.

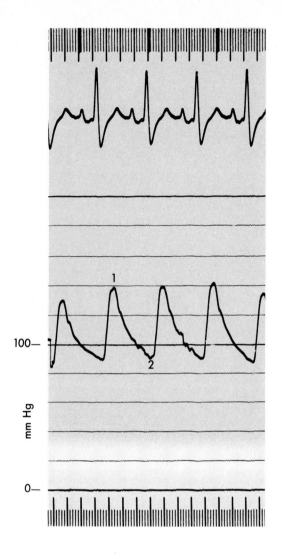

FIGURE 6-31

ANALYSIS

Rhythm: NSR

Pressure(s): Femoral artery

Waveform characteristics and measurements:

1.	Systolic	;	128	mm Hg
2.	Diastolic	;	90	mm Hg
3.		;		mm Hg
4.		;		mm Hg
5.		;		mm Hg
6.		;		mm Hg
7.		;		mm Hg

Suspected abnormality/diagnosis: Normal femoral artery pressure

Comments: The poorly defined dicrotic notch on this arterial waveform is seen commonly in the femoral artery and, thus, represents a normal variation.

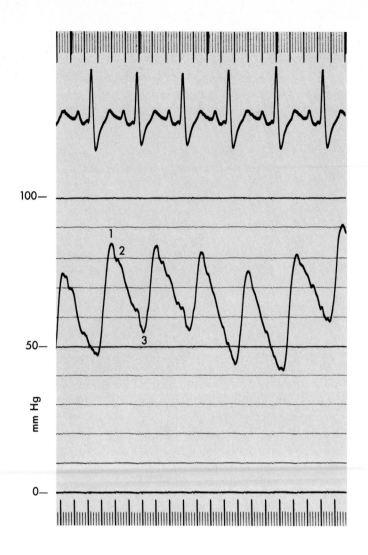

FIGURE 6-32

ANALYSIS

Rhythm: NSR

Pressure(s): PA

Waveform characteristics and measurements:

1.	Systolic	;	82	mm Hg
2.	Dicrotic notch	;		mm Hg
3.	End-diastolic	;	52	mm Hg
4.		;		mm Hg
5.		;		mm Hg
6.		;		mm Hg
7.		;		mm Hg

Suspected abnormality/diagnosis: Severe pulmonary hypertension secondary to LV failure and mitral regurgitation

Comments: This elevated PA pressure is due to severe LV failure with increased mitral regurgitation resulting in pulmonary edema.

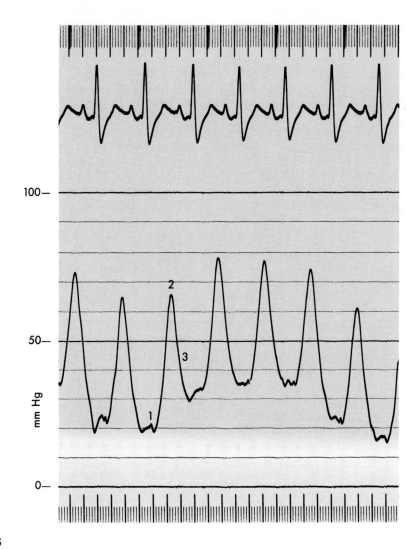

FIGURE 6-33

ANALYSIS

Rhythm: NSR

Pressure(s): PAW

Waveform characteristics and measurements:

1.	*a* Wave	;	26	mm Hg
2.	*v* Wave	;	70	mm Hg
3.	*y* Descent	;		mm Hg
4.		;		mm Hg
5.		;		mm Hg
6.		;		mm Hg
7.		;		mm Hg

Suspected abnormality/diagnosis: LV failure with severe mitral regurgitation

Comments: The elevated *a* wave of 26 mm Hg indicates LV failure while the early, dominant *v* wave is indicative of severe mitral regurgitation with subsequent signs and symptoms of congestive heart failure.

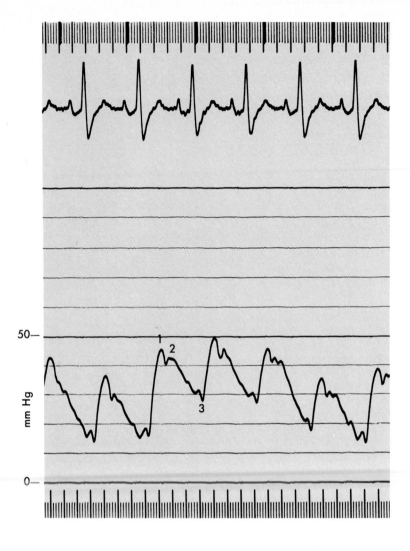

FIGURE 6-34

ANALYSIS

Rhythm: NSR

Pressure(s): PA

Waveform characteristics and measurements:

1.	Systolic	;	42	mm Hg
2.	Dicrotic notch	;		mm Hg
3.	Diastolic	;	21	mm Hg
4.		;		mm Hg
5.		;		mm Hg
6.		;		mm Hg
7.		;		mm Hg

Suspected abnormality/diagnosis: Mild LV failure with mitral regurgitation

Comments: This PA pressure has been markedly reduced as a result of both the Lasix and nitroglycerine therapy which reduced the patient's preload as well as regurgitant fraction. Note the double-humped appearance of the dicrotic notch on the fifth and sixth waveforms. This represents a retrogradely reflected v wave of approximately 35 mm Hg which is, also, markedly reduced from the previously measured v wave of 65 mm Hg.

Patient Profile 8

A 71-year-old man was admitted to the intensive care unit (ICU) following aortic valve replacement and coronary artery bypass graft to the left anterior descending (LAD) coronary artery. A PA catheter, a radial artery catheter, and a temporary pacemaker wire were placed at the time of surgery. Postoperatively, he developed complete heart block, and the pacemaker was turned on at a rate of 70 BPM. The following hemodynamic pressure waveforms were obtained (Figures 6-35 to 6-37).

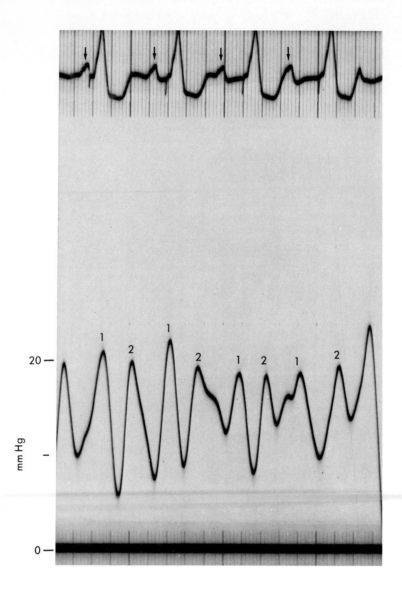

FIGURE 6-35
====

ANALYSIS

Rhythm: Paced at 70 BPM (Note pacemaker spikes and P waves in ECG.)

Pressure(s): RA

Waveform characteristics and measurements:

1.	*a* Waves	;	20	mm Hg
2.	*v* Waves	;	20	mm Hg
3.	Mean	;	15	mm Hg
4.		;		mm Hg
5.		;		mm Hg
6.		;		mm Hg
7.		;		mm Hg

Suspected abnormality/diagnosis: Hypervolemia

Comments: Note the RA *a* waves corresponding to the appearance of P waves *(arrows)* in the ECG. Note also the prominent *a* and *v* waves with rapid *x* and *y* descent, which may be due to a noncompliant RA and RV following anesthesia.

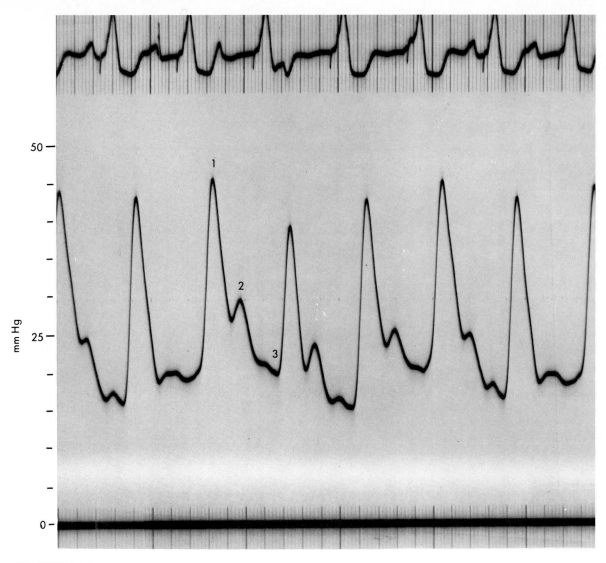

FIGURE 6-36

ANALYSIS

Rhythm: Paced at 70 BPM (Note pacemaker spikes and P waves in ECG.)

Pressure(s): PA

Waveform characteristics and measurements:

1.	PA systolic	;	42	mm Hg
2.	Dicrotic notch	;		mm Hg
3.	PA end-diastolic	;	20	mm Hg
4.		;		mm Hg
5.		;		mm Hg
6.		;		mm Hg
7.		;		mm Hg

Suspected abnormality/diagnosis: Pulmonary hypertension secondary to LV failure

Comments: The elevated PA pressure with an end-diastolic pressure of 20 mm Hg suggests congestive heart failure and the need for careful diuresis.

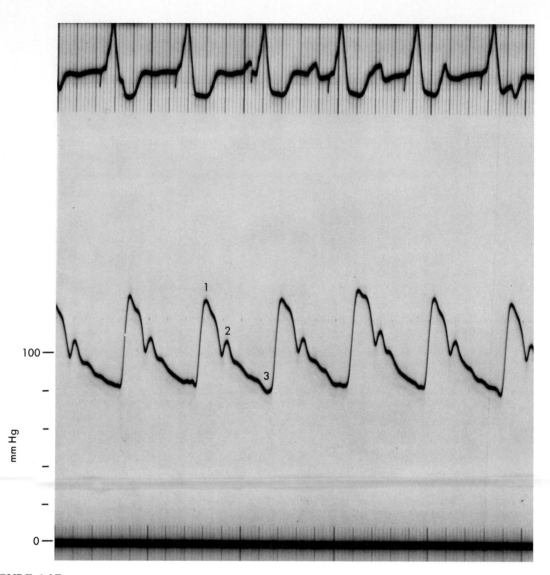

FIGURE 6-37

ANALYSIS

Rhythm: Paced at 70 BPM (Note pacemaker spikes and P waves appearing in ECG.)

Pressure(s): Radial artery

Waveform characteristics and measurements:

1.	Arterial systolic	;	112	mm Hg
2.	Dicrotic notch	;		mm Hg
3.	Arterial diastolic	;	90	mm Hg
4.		;		mm Hg
5.		;		mm Hg
6.		;		mm Hg
7.		;		mm Hg

Suspected abnormality/diagnosis: Normal arterial pressure

Comments:

156

Patient Profile 9

A 30-year-old man was admitted to the CCU with complaints of dyspnea on exertion and the occurrence of blackout spells during exercise. Prior cardiac catheterization confirmed the diagnosis of severe primary pulmonary hypertension. Hemodynamic instrumentation was instituted to evaluate his hemodynamic response to a trial of vasodilator therapy in an attempt to control his pulmonary hypertension. Unfortunately, as the following pressure tracings illustrate (Figures 6-38 to 6-43), this patient's pulmonary hypertension was very severe and resistant to vasodilator therapy, including nitroprusside and isoproterenol, making him a candidate for heart-lung transplantation.

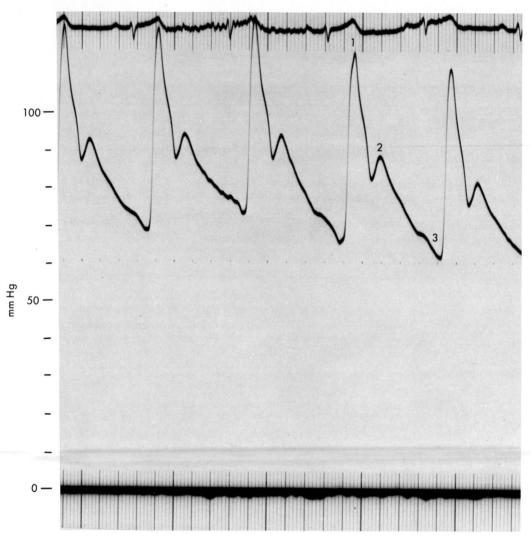

FIGURE 6-38

ANALYSIS

Rhythm: NSR
Pressure(s): PA
Waveform characteristics and measurements:

1.	PA systolic	;	119	mm Hg
2.	Dicrotic notch	;		mm Hg
3.	PA end-diastolic	;	65	mm Hg
4.		;		mm Hg
5.		;		mm Hg
6.		;		mm Hg
7.		;		mm Hg

Suspected abnormality/diagnosis: Severe pulmonary hypertension
Comments:

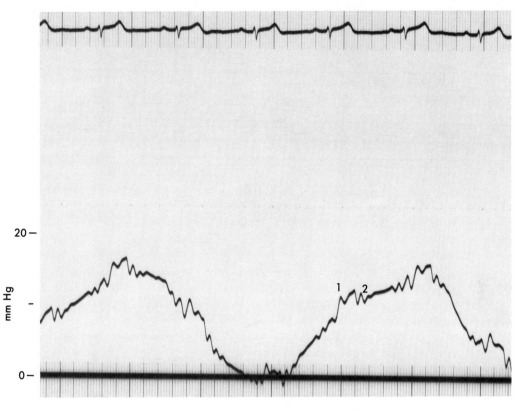

FIGURE 6-39

ANALYSIS

Rhythm: NSR

Pressure(s): PAW

Waveform characteristics and measurements:

1.	*a* Wave	;	mm Hg
2.	*v* Wave	;	mm Hg
3.	Mean	; 10	mm Hg
4.		;	mm Hg
5.		;	mm Hg
6.		;	mm Hg
7.		;	mm Hg

Suspected abnormality/diagnosis: Normal PAW

Comments: Exaggerated respiratory changes make exact identification of the *a* and *v* waves difficult. That exact an identification is not necessary, however, since neither the *a* nor the *v* wave is particularly dominant or elevated. In this case a mean PAW pressure, which averages the pressure changes during one complete respiratory cycle, more closely reflects the LVedp. Such exaggerated respiratory changes are commonly seen in patients with pulmonary hypertension. The normal mean value of this PAW pressure precludes LV dysfunction as the cause of this patient's pulmonary hypertension.

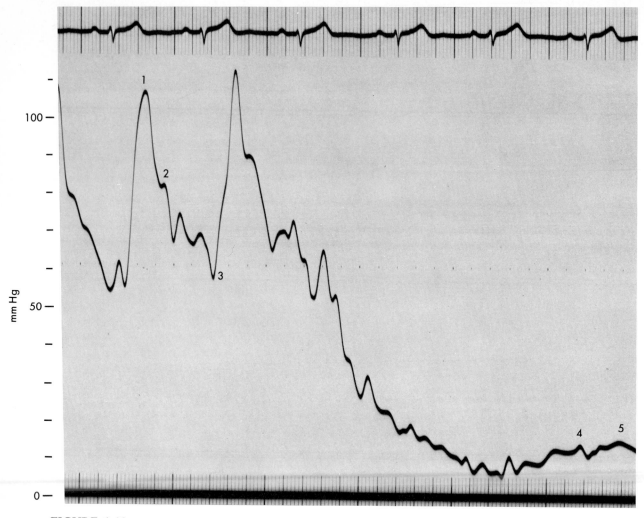

FIGURE 6-40

ANALYSIS

Rhythm: NSR

Pressure(s): PA to PAW

Waveform characteristics and measurements:

1.	PA systolic	;	108	mm Hg
2.	Dicrotic notch	;		mm Hg
3.	PA end-diastolic	;	55	mm Hg
4.	PAW *a* wave	;	10	mm Hg
5.	PAW *v* wave	;	10	mm Hg
6.		;		mm Hg
7.		;		mm Hg

Suspected abnormality/diagnosis: Severe primary pulmonary hypertension

Comments: The extremely high PA pressure (108/55) with normal PAW pressures reflects a high PVR due to pulmonary vascular disease. Left heart failure can be ruled out as the cause in the presence of a normal PAW pressure of 10 mm Hg. In this case the PA pressure does not reflect the LVedp but, rather, the high PVR. Preload of the left ventricle can still be monitored, however, through measurement of the PAW pressure. This shows the importance of obtaining an initial correlation between the PAedp and PA pressures before using the PAedp to monitor the LVedp. In this case, only the PAW pressure can be used to monitor LV preload.

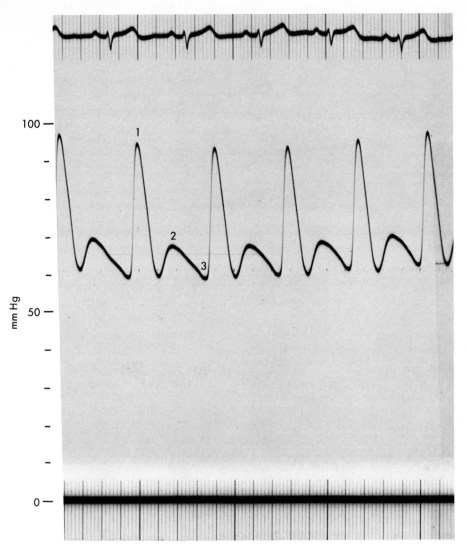

FIGURE 6-41

ANALYSIS

Rhythm: NSR

Pressure(s): Radial artery

Waveform characteristics and measurements:

1.	Arterial systolic	;	97	mm Hg
2.	Dicrotic notch	;		mm Hg
3.	Arterial diastolic	;	60	mm Hg
4.		;		mm Hg
5.		;		mm Hg
6.		;		mm Hg
7.		;		mm Hg

Suspected abnormality/diagnosis: Hypotension secondary to afterload reduction

Comments: This is the arterial pressure during nitroprusside therapy, reflecting a decrease in systolic pressure, enhanced, rapid ejection during systole, and rapid runoff during diastole.

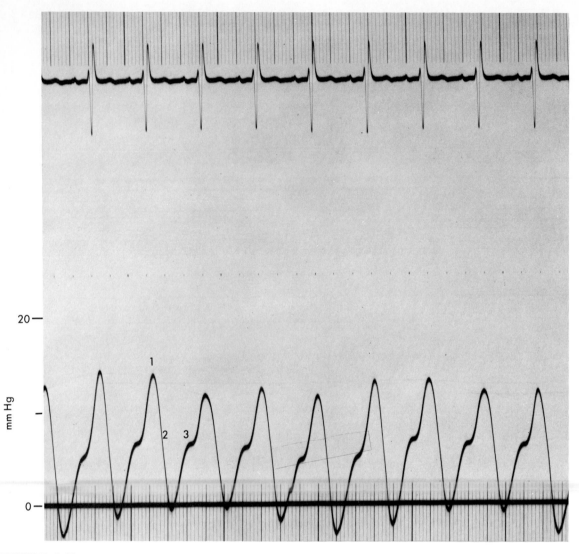

FIGURE 6-42

ANALYSIS

Rhythm: NSR (sensitivity increased)

Pressure(s): RA

Waveform characteristics and measurements:

1.		*a* Wave	;	12	mm Hg
2.		*x* Descent	;		mm Hg
3.		*v* Wave	;	7	mm Hg
4.		Mean	;	6	mm Hg
5.			;		mm Hg
6.			;		mm Hg
7.			;		mm Hg

Suspected abnormality/diagnosis: RV failure

Comments: This RA pressure tracing was taken 24 hours later and shows a prominent *a* wave and *x* descent. This is due to hypertrophy of the RV secondary to pulmonary hypertension and high PVR.

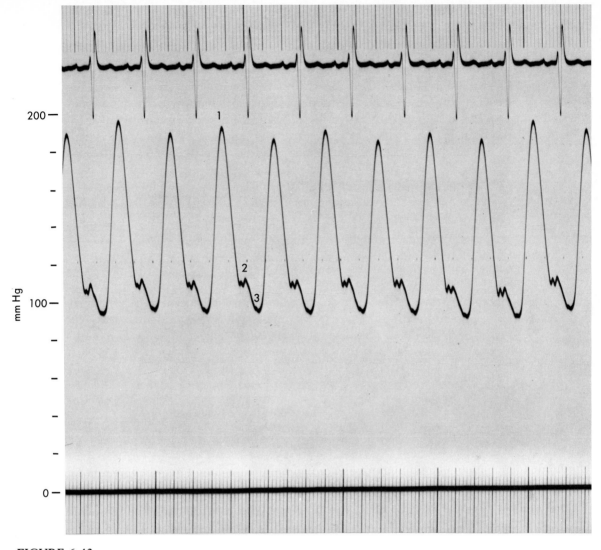

FIGURE 6-43

ANALYSIS

Rhythm: Sinus tachycardia

Pressure(s): PA

Waveform characteristics and measurements:

1.	PA systolic	;	195	mm Hg
2.	Dicrotic notch	;		mm Hg
3.	PA end-diastolic	;	95	mm Hg
4.		;		mm Hg
5.		;		mm Hg
6.		;		mm Hg
7.		;		mm Hg

Suspected abnormality/diagnosis: Severe pulmonary hypertension unresponsive to isoproterenol infusion

Comments: This PA pressure tracing was obtained 24 hours after that in Figure 6-38 and during an infusion of isoproterenol in an attempt to reduce PVR and the PA pressure. Unfortunately the desired effect was not achieved, and the PA pressure rose even higher, prompting immediate cessation of isoproterenol administration.

A 54-year-old woman underwent mitral valvuloplasty for severe mitral stenosis secondary to rheumatic fever. The patient had been in atrial fibrillation for 3 years and was receiving Coumadin (2.5 mg/day). Three days before undergoing an elective mitral valvuloplasty the Coumadin was discontinued and systemic heparinization was begun to prevent embolization. Mitral valvuloplasty was performed using the transseptal approach. The mitral valve was dilated 3 times with a 15 mm and 20 mm balloon combination, and 3 times with an 18 mm and 20 mm balloon combination. Evidence of waisting was not present at the last inflation, and repeat hemodynamics revealed a decrease in the mitral valve gradient from 13 to 6 mm Hg with an increase in mitral valve area from 0.4 to 0.94 cm^2. The patient tolerated the procedure well and returned to the CCU with a sheath in the femoral artery and a PA catheter in place.

Approximately 30 minutes after her return, the patient's heart rate rose from the 80s to approximately 120 to 130 beats/min. The following hemodynamic pressures were obtained at that time (Figures 6-44 to 6-46).

A chest x-ray showed an increase in the cardiac border and an emergency echocardiogram confirmed the presence of pericardial effusion. Emergent pericardiocentesis was performed with removal of approximately 450 ml of blood. The hemodynamic pressure in Figure 6-47 was obtained immediately following pericardiocentesis.

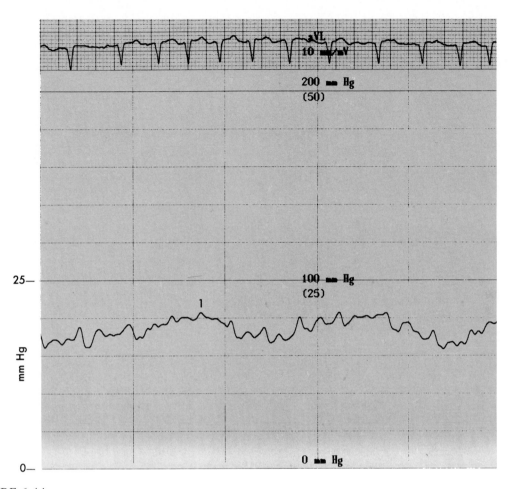

FIGURE 6-44

ANALYSIS

Rhythm: Atrial fibrillation with rapid ventricular response

Pressure(s): RA

Waveform characteristics and measurements:

1.	*v* Wave	; 17	mm Hg
2.	Mean	; 17	mm Hg
3.		;	mm Hg
4.		;	mm Hg
5.		;	mm Hg
6.		;	mm Hg
7.		;	mm Hg

Suspected abnormality/diagnosis: Cardiac tamponade

Comments: Because of the underlying atrial fibrillation, there is no *a* wave present in this RA waveform. This rhythm also obviates the classical RA waveform associated with tamponade, that is, a normal *x* descent with a very brief *y* descent. The elevated mean RA pressure of 17 mm Hg suggests right heart dysfunction.

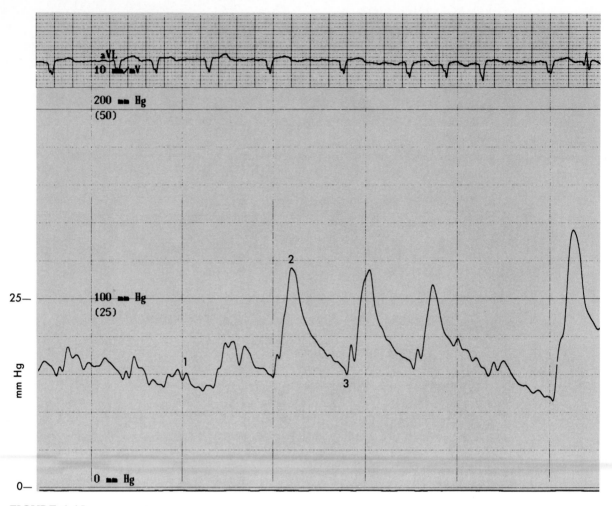

FIGURE 6-45

ANALYSIS

Rhythm: Atrial fibrillation

Pressure(s): PAW/PA

Waveform characteristics and measurements:

#				
1.	PAW *v* Wave	;	16	mm Hg
2.	PA systolic	;	27	mm Hg
3.	PA diastolic	;	16	mm Hg
4.		;		mm Hg
5.		;		mm Hg
6.		;		mm Hg
7.		;		mm Hg

Suspected abnormality/diagnosis: Cardiac tamponade

Comments: The slightly elevated PAW mean pressure of 16 mm Hg is due to residual mitral stenosis. Note the similarity between the preceding RA mean pressure (Figure 6-44) and the mean PAW and PA end-diastolic pressures above. This equalization of pressures is seen in cardiac tamponade where there is restriction during all of diastole.

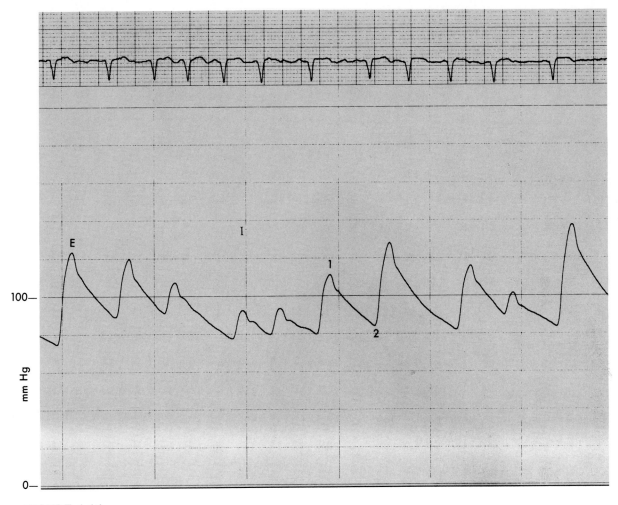

FIGURE 6-46

ANALYSIS

Rhythm: Atrial fibrillation

Pressure(s): Radial artery

Waveform characteristics and measurements:

1.	Systolic	;	96-124	mm Hg
2.	Diastolic	;	80-90	mm Hg
3.		;		mm Hg
4.		;		mm Hg
5.		;		mm Hg
6.		;		mm Hg
7.		;		mm Hg

Suspected abnormality/diagnosis: Cardiac tamponade

Comments: The 25 mm Hg drop in arterial systolic pressure during spontaneous inhalation *(I)* is termed pulsus paradoxus and is seen, classically, in patients with cardiac tamponade with further declines in stroke volume during inspiration.

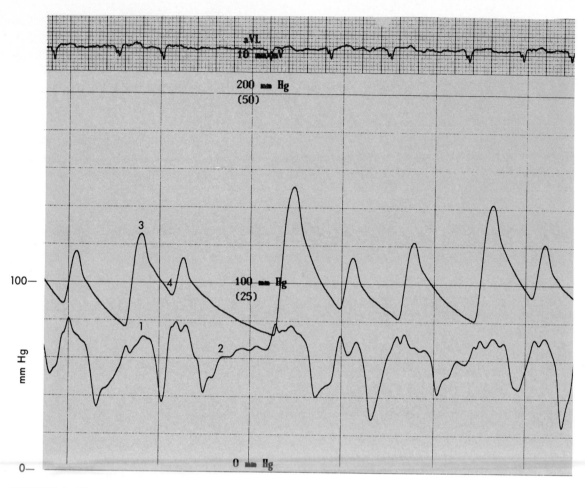

FIGURE 6-47

ANALYSIS

Rhythm: Atrial fibrillation
Pressure(s): Radial artery and RA
Waveform characteristics and measurements:

1.	RA v wave	;	17	mm Hg
2.	RA mean	;	13	mm Hg
3.	Arterial systolic	;	130	mm Hg
4.	Arterial diastolic	;	80	mm Hg
5.		;		mm Hg
6.		;		mm Hg
7.		;		mm Hg

Suspected abnormality/diagnosis: Post-pericardiocentesis hemodynamics with mild right heart overload

Comments: While the RA pressure post-pericardiocentesis remains moderately elevated, its contour is normal for the cardiac rhythm and is similar to the pretamponade pressure contour and value. The variation in arterial systolic pressure is now due to varying RR intervals and not associated with respiratory changes.

168

Patient Profile 11

A 45-year-old male was admitted with a 2-week history of a 20-lb weight gain, decreased appetite, early satiety, peripheral edema, and severe shortness of breath (SOB). The patient also complained of sharp pain in the right upper quadrant (RUO) of the abdomen. Past medical history included hospitalization 1 year ago for both pericardial and pleural effusion of unknown etiology although viral titers were positive for both coxsackie and echovirus. He was also noted to have hepatitis A and B antibodies at that time.

The patient's blood pressure was 100/70, heart rate was 92 beats/min, and respiratory rate was 20 breaths/min. Jugular venous distention was present to the angle of the jaw with a suggestion of Kussmaul's sign. Crackles were present at the bases of both lungs.

Cardiovascular exam revealed an indistinct PMI, a normal S_1 and S_2, and the presence of an S_4 with a loud pericardial rub heard at the apex.

The patient's abdomen was markedly distended, the liver was enlarged, and 1+ peripheral edema was present. To determine if LV failure was present in addition to assessing the extent of RV failure, a PA catheter was inserted and the following hemodynamic pressures obtained (Figures 6-48 to 6-53).

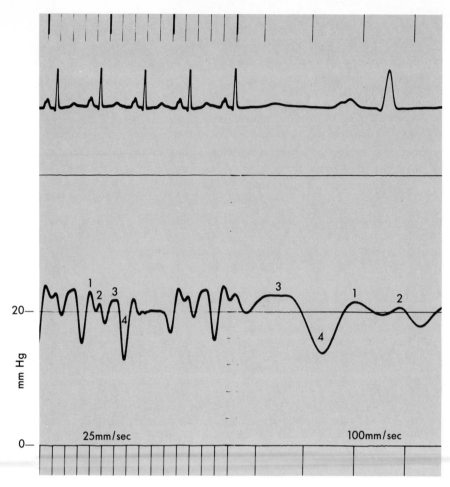

20—

mm Hg

0—

25mm/sec   100mm/sec

FIGURE 6-48

ANALYSIS

Rhythm: NSR

Pressure(s): RA

Waveform characteristics and measurements:

1.	*a* wave	; 22	mm Hg
2.	*c* Wave	;	mm Hg
3.	*v* Wave	; 22	mm Hg
4.	*y* Descent	;	mm Hg
5.		;	mm Hg
6.		;	mm Hg
7.		;	mm Hg

Suspected abnormality/diagnosis: Constrictive pericarditis

Comments: Both the *a* and *v* waves are equally elevated in this RA pressure, however, the *y* descent is exaggerated and dominant. This feature is typically associated with constrictive pericarditis and is due to the rapid, early filling during the beginning of diastole which is abruptly halted when the constraints of the rigid pericardium are suddenly met.

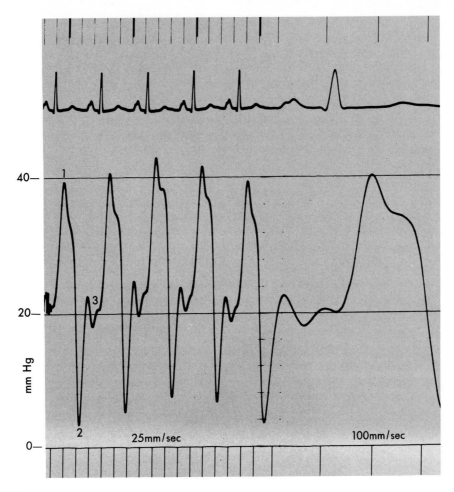

FIGURE 6-49

ANALYSIS

Rhythm: NSR

Pressure(s): RV

Waveform characteristics and measurements:

1.	Systolic	; 40	mm Hg
2.	Diastolic	; 4	mm Hg
3.	End-diastolic	; 22	mm Hg
4.		;	mm Hg
5.		;	mm Hg
6.		;	mm Hg
7.		;	mm Hg

Suspected abnormality/diagnosis: Constrictive pericarditis

Comments: This RV pressure, obtained as the catheter passes through the right heart, is markedly elevated and reveals a "square root" pattern during diastole, again, reflecting the rapid ventricular filling during early diastole until the constricted pericardium suddenly prevents further filling. Note the similarity between the RV end-diastolic pressure and the preceding RA mean pressure (Figure 6-48).

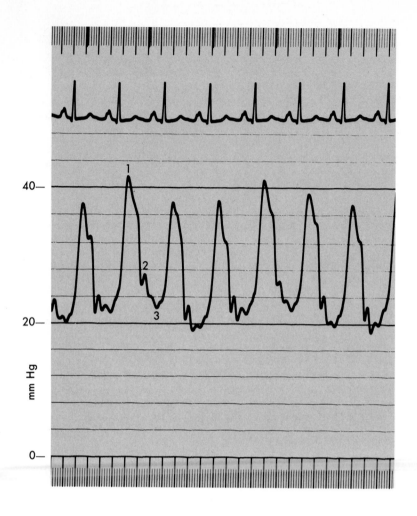

FIGURE 6-50

ANALYSIS

Rhythm: NSR

Pressure(s): PA

Waveform characteristics and measurements:

1.	Systolic	;	39	mm Hg
2.	Dicrotic notch	;		mm Hg
3.	Diastolic	;	22	mm Hg
4.		;		mm Hg
5.		;		mm Hg
6.		;		mm Hg
7.		;		mm Hg

Suspected abnormality/diagnosis: Constrictive pericarditis

Comments: Note the elevated diastolic pressure of 22 mm Hg is the same as the preceding RA and RV end-diastolic pressures (Figures 6-48 and 6-49) representing equalization of pressures due to pericardial constriction of the entire heart.

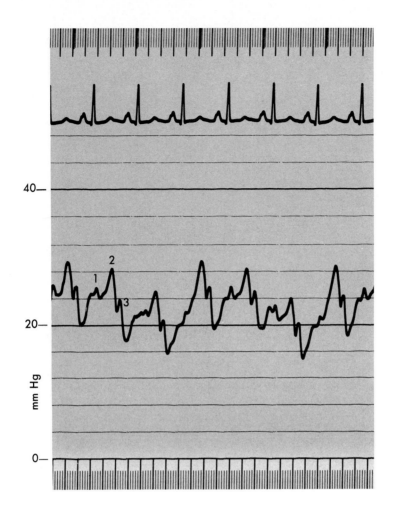

FIGURE 6-51

ANALYSIS

Rhythm: NSR

Pressure(s): PAW

Waveform characteristics and measurements:

1.	*a* Wave	;	22	mm Hg
2.	*v* Wave	;	26	mm Hg
3.	*y* Descent	;		mm Hg
4.	Mean	;	23	mm Hg
5.		;		mm Hg
6.		;		mm Hg
7.		;		mm Hg

Suspected abnormality/diagnosis: Constrictive pericarditis

Comments: Note the similarity between the mean PAW pressure of 23 mm Hg and the previous RA mean, RV end-diastolic and PA end-diastolic pressures (Figures 6-48 to 6-50).

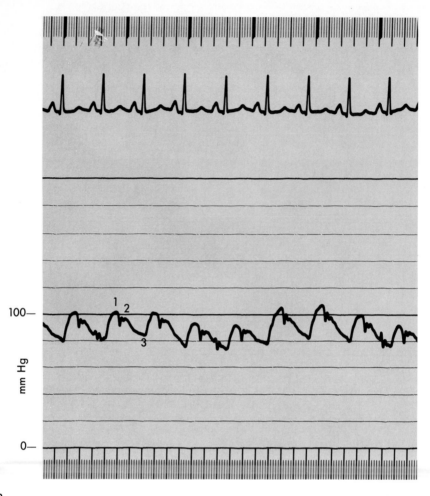

FIGURE 6-52

ANALYSIS

Rhythm: NSR

Pressure(s): Radial artery

Waveform characteristics and measurements:

1.	Systolic	;	100	mm Hg
2.	Dicrotic notch	;		mm Hg
3.	Diastole	;	80	mm Hg
4.		;		mm Hg
5.		;		mm Hg
6.		;		mm Hg
7.		;		mm Hg

Suspected abnormality/diagnosis: Hypotension associated with constrictive pericarditis

Comments: The small pulse pressure (20 mm Hg) of this arterial pressure reflects the diminished stroke volume as a result of the constrictive pericarditis.

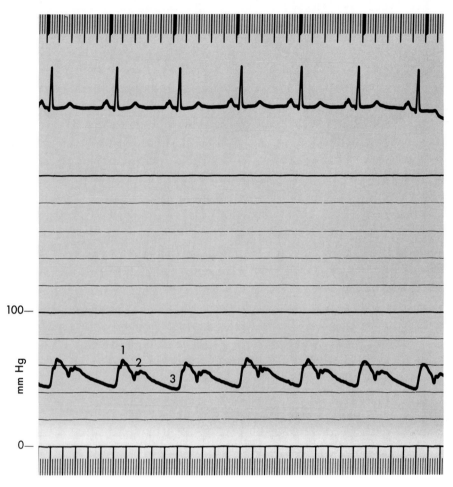

FIGURE 6-53

ANALYSIS

Rhythm: Sinus bradycardia

Pressure(s): Radial artery

Waveform characteristics and measurements:

1.	Systolic	;	60	mm Hg
2.	Dicrotic notch	;		mm Hg
3.	Diastole	;	45	mm Hg
4.		;		mm Hg
5.		;		mm Hg
6.		;		mm Hg
7.		;		mm Hg

Suspected abnormality/diagnosis: Severe hypotension secondary to vasovagal reaction

Comments: This severely reduced arterial pressure is associated with a vasovagal reaction (note the slower heart rate) which was successfully treated with atropine and volume administration.

Chapter 7

Self-Assessment

This section consists of numerous and varied hemodynamic pressure tracings for the reader to assess his or her skill in identifying and interpreting both normal and abnormal pressure waveforms.

A systematic approach to identification of pressure waveforms is most useful. The following steps offer one method of waveform analysis. However, whatever method is used, consistently answering the following questions can minimize confusion.

1. What is the cardiac rhythm?

Knowledge of the patient's heart rhythm offers clues as to what to look for in the pressure waveform. With atrial fibrillation the atrial pressures (RA, LA, or PAW) will reveal only a *v* wave after each QRS complex. In AV dissociation it is possible to see unusually large cannon *a* waves in the atrial pressure waveform. The arterial pressure contour (either pulmonary artery or systemic artery), in atrial fibrillation, will exhibit marked variation in pulse pressure.

2. What type of waveform does it look like?

By this time, having seen numerous normal waveforms, you know what atrial pressures (RA, LA, and PAW), ventricular pressures, or arterial pressures look like. The answer to this question may be: "This pressure looks like what I know an atrial pressure looks like. I see a low pressure with an *a* wave and a *v* wave." Or it may be: "This looks like an arterial type of pressure with an upstroke, systole, dicrotic notch, and diastole." Or: "This pressure looks like a ventricular pressure with the systolic pressure the same as the PA systolic pressure, but the diastolic pressure falling down to baseline."

3. Is the contour of the pressure waveform normal?

Having identified the pressure, it is important to note if the contour or the characteristics of the pressure waveform are normal. With the atrial pressure, is either the *a* or the *v* wave dominant? Is either the *x* or *y* descent prominent or abbreviated? With the arterial pressures (PA or systemic arterial), is the upstroke rapid or slow? Is the dicrotic notch present or absent? Is the runoff period prolonged or abbreviated?

4. Is the value of the pressure waveform normal?

Having identified the pressure and assessed its characteristics, it is important to measure the value of the pressure and determine whether it falls within normal ranges. Look carefully at the value scale indicated on the left side of the tracing. With the atrial pressures (RA, LA, or PAW), a mean or average pressure is usually recorded. However, if the *v* wave is particularly dominant and elevated, both the *a* and *v* waves should be measured and recorded. In the following tracings, you should indicate the values of both *a* and *v* waves. It is not necessary, however, to note the value of the *c* wave, even though you are asked to identify it. With the arterial pressure (PA and systemic arterial), the systolic, diastolic, and mean values are recorded. It is not necessary to note the value of the dicrotic notch, only to identify its presence or absence.

A cautionary note regarding "normal values" must be mentioned here. The values of the hemodynamic pressures must always be correlated with the patient's clinical picture! For example, even though a mean PAW pressure of 8 mm Hg may be normal in one clinical setting, it may be abnormally low for the patient with a low cardiac output. No single hemodynamic parameter or measurement should be used to guide medical care.

5. What is the suspected abnormality?

Based on the answers to the four previous questions, it should be possible to reach some answer regarding possible pathophysiology. Hemodynamic data can provide information regarding some cardiac abnormalities, but they are usually not used to provide definitive diagnosis. This usually requires more extensive information obtained from echocardiography and cardiac catheterization.

In the following pressures you are asked to identify, there could be one or more pathologic conditions responsible for the pressure abnormalities. To avoid repetition, only the more likely abnormality is listed, although you may be correct in listing others.

One last word of caution before proceeding with the pressure waveform identification. Frequently there occur many small, regular and consistent pressure rises in hemodynamic pressure tracings. These pressure rises or oscillations are hemodynamically insignificant. Too often, having learned to identify the pressure characteristics of certain waveforms, there is a tendency to place emphasis on every little oscillation in the pressure waveform.

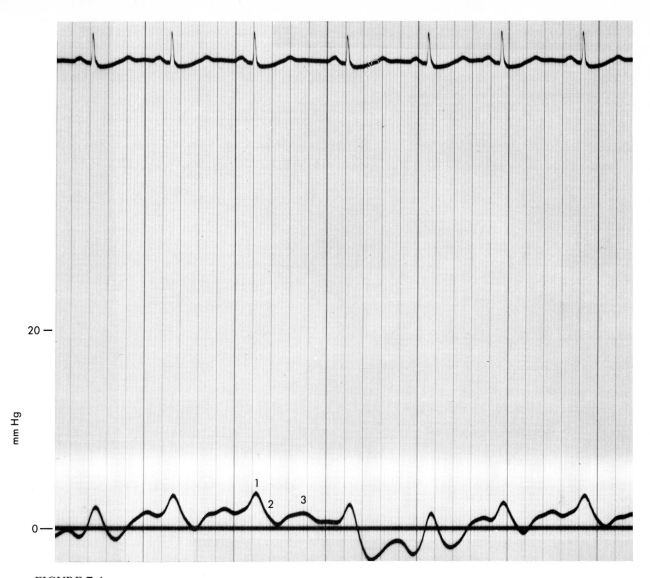

FIGURE 7-1

ANALYSIS

Rhythm:

Pressure(s):

Waveform characteristics and measurements:

1. _____ ; _____ mm Hg
2. _____ ; _____ mm Hg
3. _____ ; _____ mm Hg
4. _____ ; _____ mm Hg
5. _____ ; _____ mm Hg
6. _____ ; _____ mm Hg
7. _____ ; _____ mm Hg

Suspected abnormality/diagnosis:

Comments:

ANALYSIS of Figure 7-1

Rhythm: NSR

Pressure(s): RA

Waveform characteristics and measurements:

1.	*a* Wave	;	3	mm Hg
2.	*x* Descent	;		mm Hg
3.	*v* Wave	;	1	mm Hg
4.	Mean	;	0-1	mm Hg
5.		;		mm Hg
6.		;		mm Hg
7.		;		mm Hg

Suspected abnormality/diagnosis: Hypovolemia or inaccurate placement of transducer air-reference level above level of RA

Comments: The normal fall in RA pressure during inspiration becomes negative in this abnormally low RA pressure.

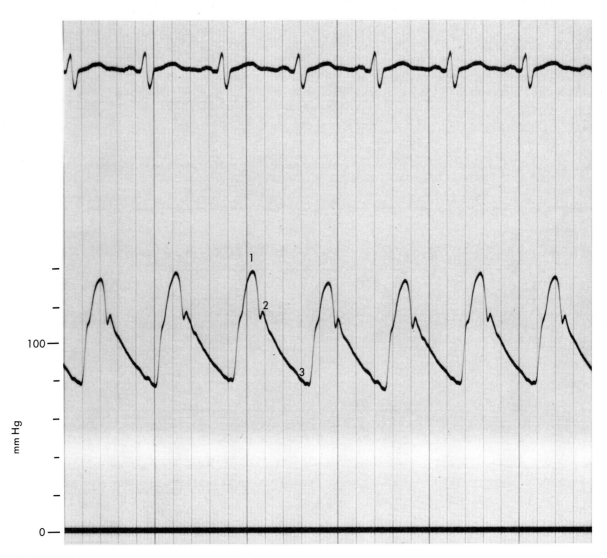

FIGURE 7-2

ANALYSIS

Rhythm:

Pressure(s):

Waveform characteristics and measurements:

1. _____ ; _____ mm Hg
2. _____ ; _____ mm Hg
3. _____ ; _____ mm Hg
4. _____ ; _____ mm Hg
5. _____ ; _____ mm Hg
6. _____ ; _____ mm Hg
7. _____ ; _____ mm Hg

Suspected abnormality/diagnosis:

Comments:

ANALYSIS of Figure 7-2

Rhythm: NSR

Pressure(s): Radial artery

Waveform characteristics and measurements:

1.	Arterial systolic	;	135	mm Hg
2.	Dicrotic notch	;		mm Hg
3.	Arterial end-diastolic	;	75	mm Hg
4.		;		mm Hg
5.		;		mm Hg
6.		;		mm Hg
7.		;		mm Hg

Suspected abnormality/diagnosis: Normal arterial pressure

Comments:

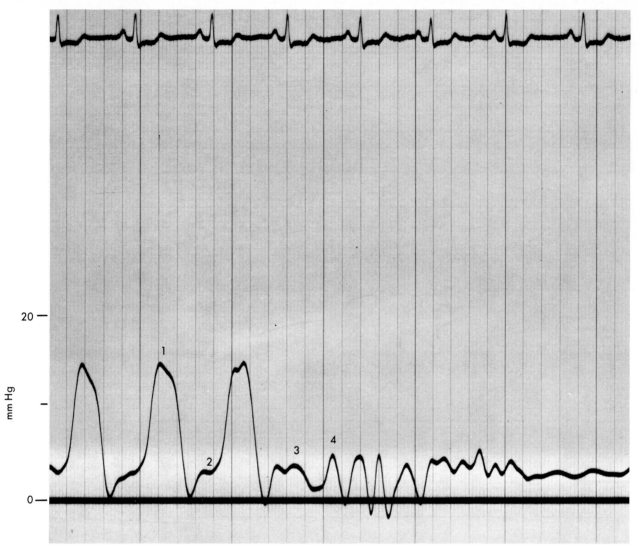

FIGURE 7-3

ANALYSIS

Rhythm:

Pressure(s):

Waveform characteristics and measurements:

1. _____ ; _____ mm Hg
2. _____ ; _____ mm Hg
3. _____ ; _____ mm Hg
4. _____ ; _____ mm Hg
5. _____ ; _____ mm Hg
6. _____ ; _____ mm Hg
7. _____ ; _____ mm Hg

Suspected abnormality/diagnosis:

Comments:

ANALYSIS of Figure 7-3

Rhythm: NSR

Pressure(s): RV to RA

Waveform characteristics and measurements:

1.	RV systolic	;	15	mm Hg
2.	RV end-diastolic	;	4	mm Hg
3.	RA *a* wave	;	4	mm Hg
4.	RA *v* wave	;	5	mm Hg
5.	RA mean	;	4	mm Hg
6.		;		mm Hg
7.		;		mm Hg

Suspected abnormality/diagnosis: Normal

Comments: The catheter is withdrawn from the RV into the RA. The RA pressure waveform becomes damped, most likely because of curling of the catheter in the RA and pushing of the catheter tip against the atrial wall. When the catheter is resting in the PA, it forms a distinct curve. Frequently this curve is maintained, even when the catheter is withdrawn into another chamber.

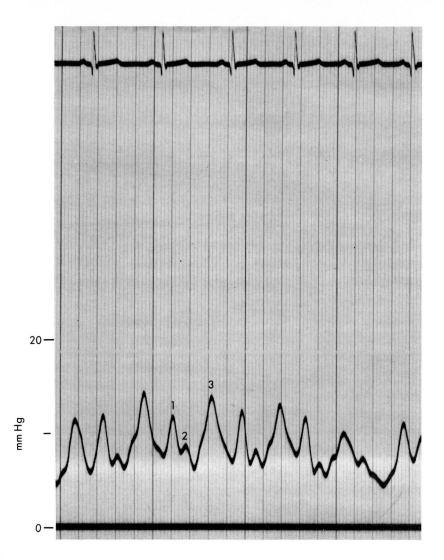

FIGURE 7-4

ANALYSIS

Rhythm:

Pressure(s):

Waveform characteristics and measurements:

1. _____ ; _____ mm Hg
2. _____ ; _____ mm Hg
3. _____ ; _____ mm Hg
4. _____ ; _____ mm Hg
5. _____ ; _____ mm Hg
6. _____ ; _____ mm Hg
7. _____ ; _____ mm Hg

Suspected abnormality/diagnosis:

Comments:

ANALYSIS of Figure 7-4

Rhythm: NSR

Pressure(s): PAW

Waveform characteristics and measurements:

1.	*a* Wave	;	12	mm Hg
2.	*c* Wave	;		mm Hg
3.	*v* wave	;	13	mm Hg
4.	Mean	;	9	mm Hg
5.		;		mm Hg
6.		;		mm Hg
7.		;		mm Hg

Suspected abnormality/diagnosis: Normal PAW pressure

Comments:

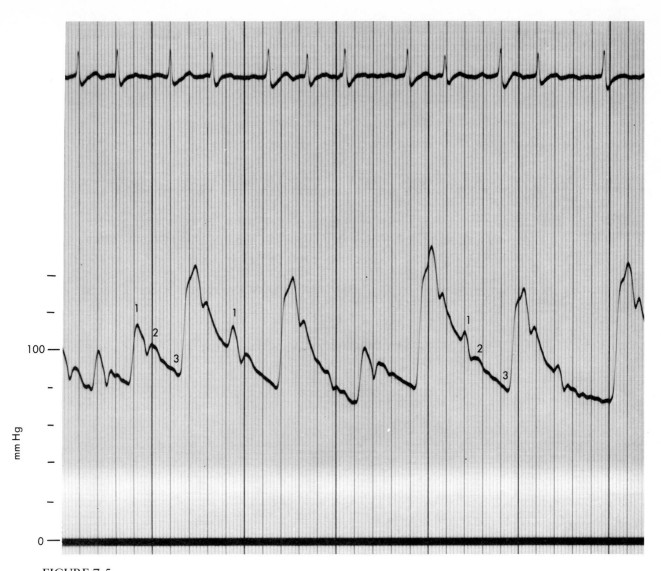

FIGURE 7-5

ANALYSIS

Rhythm:

Pressure(s):

Waveform characteristics and measurements:

1. _____ ; _____ mm Hg
2. _____ ; _____ mm Hg
3. _____ ; _____ mm Hg
4. _____ ; _____ mm Hg
5. _____ ; _____ mm Hg
6. _____ ; _____ mm Hg
7. _____ ; _____ mm Hg

Suspected abnormality/diagnosis:

Comments:

ANALYSIS of Figure 7-5

Rhythm: Atrial fibrillation

Pressure(s): Radial artery

Waveform characteristics and measurements:

1.	Arterial systolic	;	100-145	mm Hg
2.	Dicrotic notch	;		mm Hg
3.	Arterial end-diastolic	;	78	mm Hg
4.		;		mm Hg
5.		;		mm Hg
6.		;		mm Hg
7.		;		mm Hg

Suspected abnormality/diagnosis: Normal arterial pressure

Comments: Note the marked beat-to-beat systolic pressure variation due to atrial fibrillation with varying RR intervals.

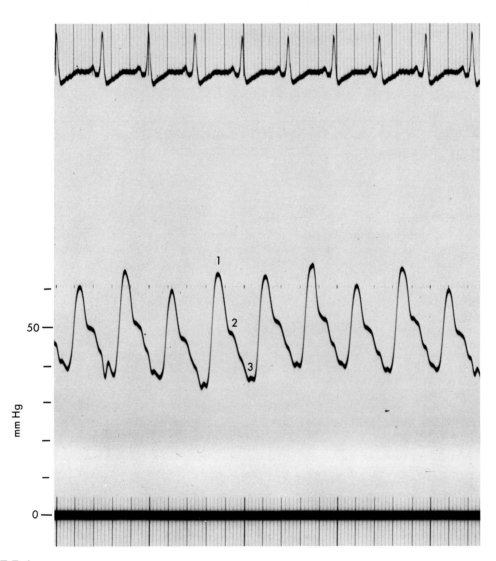

FIGURE 7-6

ANALYSIS

Rhythm:

Pressure(s):

Waveform characteristics and measurements:

1.	_____ ;	_____ mm Hg
2.	_____ ;	_____ mm Hg
3.	_____ ;	_____ mm Hg
4.	_____ ;	_____ mm Hg
5.	_____ ;	_____ mm Hg
6.	_____ ;	_____ mm Hg
7.	_____ ;	_____ mm Hg

Suspected abnormality/diagnosis:

Comments:

ANALYSIS of Figure 7-6

Rhythm: Sinus tachycardia

Pressure(s): PA

Waveform characteristics and measurements:

1.	PA systolic	;	62	mm Hg
2.	Dicrotic notch	;		mm Hg
3.	PA end-diastolic	;	38	mm Hg
4.		;		mm Hg
5.		;		mm Hg
6.		;		mm Hg
7.		;		mm Hg

Suspected abnormality/diagnosis: Pulmonary hypertension

Comments: The broadened shape of the dicrotic notch is highly suggestive of a superimposed v wave from the LA due to severe mitral regurgitation. Comparison to the PAW pressure is necessary to confirm this.

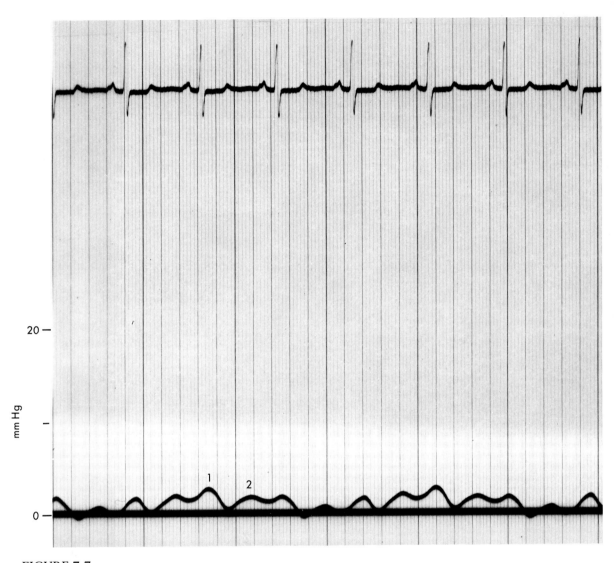

FIGURE 7-7

ANALYSIS

Rhythm:

Pressure(s):

Waveform characteristics and measurements:

1. _____ ; _____ mm Hg
2. _____ ; _____ mm Hg
3. _____ ; _____ mm Hg
4. _____ ; _____ mm Hg
5. _____ ; _____ mm Hg
6. _____ ; _____ mm Hg
7. _____ ; _____ mm Hg

Suspected abnormality/diagnosis:

Comments:

191

ANALYSIS of Figure 7-7

Rhythm: NSR

Pressure(s): PAW

Waveform characteristics and measurements:

1.	_a_ Wave	;	2	mm Hg
2.	_v_ Wave	;	1	mm Hg
3.	Mean	;	1	mm Hg
4.		;		mm Hg
5.		;		mm Hg
6.		;		mm Hg
7.		;		mm Hg

Suspected abnormality/diagnosis: Hypovolemia or incorrect transducer air-reference level placement above the level of the atria.

Comments:

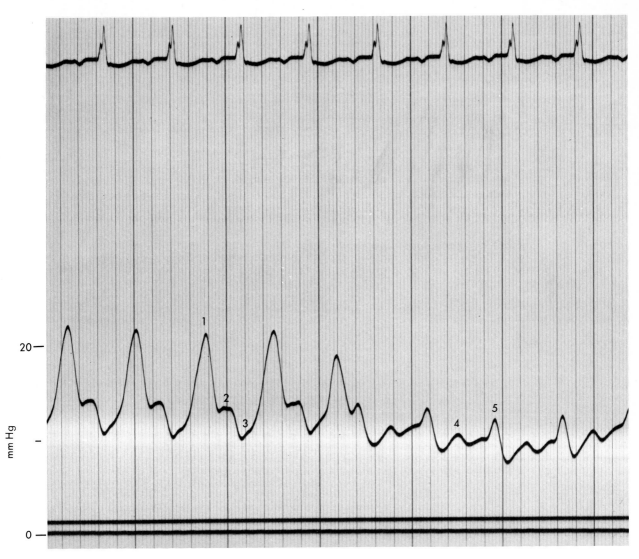

FIGURE 7-8

ANALYSIS

Rhythm:

Pressure(s):

Waveform characteristics and measurements:

1. _____ ; _____ mm Hg
2. _____ ; _____ mm Hg
3. _____ ; _____ mm Hg
4. _____ ; _____ mm Hg
5. _____ ; _____ mm Hg
6. _____ ; _____ mm Hg
7. _____ ; _____ mm Hg

Suspected abnormality/diagnosis:

Comments:

ANALYSIS of Figure 7-8

Rhythm: NSR with 1° A-V Block

Pressure(s): PA to PAW

Waveform characteristics and measurements:

1.	PA systolic	;	22	mm Hg
2.	Dicrotic notch	;		mm Hg
3.	PA end-diastolic	;	10	mm Hg
4.	PAW *a* wave	;	10	mm Hg
5.	PAW *v* wave	;	12	mm Hg
6.	PAW mean	;	10	mm Hg
7.		;		mm Hg

Suspected abnormality/diagnosis: Normal

Comments: Note the similarity between the PAW pressure and the PAedp. Since the contour of the PAW pressure waveform is normal and its value correlates closely with the PAedp, it is prudent to monitor the PAedp as a reflection of the LVedp and thus minimize the risks associated with balloon inflation.

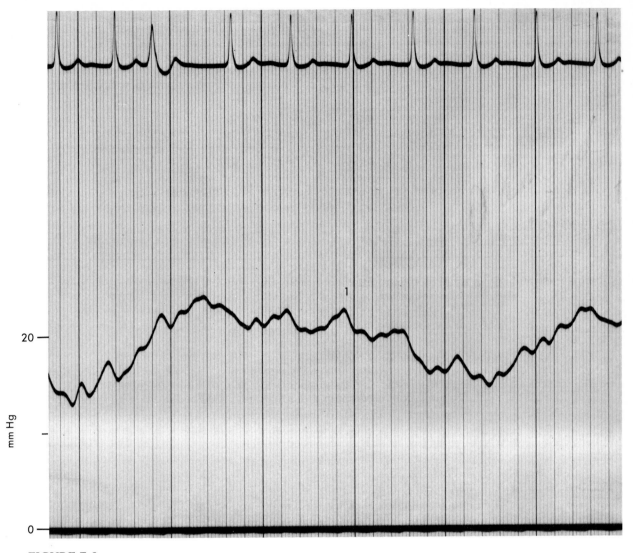

FIGURE 7-9

ANALYSIS

Rhythm:

Pressure(s):

Waveform characteristics and measurements:

1. _____ ; _____ mm Hg
2. _____ ; _____ mm Hg
3. _____ ; _____ mm Hg
4. _____ ; _____ mm Hg
5. _____ ; _____ mm Hg
6. _____ ; _____ mm Hg
7. _____ ; _____ mm Hg

Suspected abnormality/diagnosis:

Comments:

ANALYSIS of Figure 7-9

Rhythm: Atrial fibrillation with a PVC
Pressure(s): PAW
Waveform characteristics and measurements:

1. _____ _v_ Wave _____ ; _____ 19 _____ mm Hg
2. _____ Mean _____ ; _____ 19 _____ mm Hg
3. _____ ; _____ mm Hg
4. _____ ; _____ mm Hg
5. _____ ; _____ mm Hg
6. _____ ; _____ mm Hg
7. _____ ; _____ mm Hg

Suspected abnormality/diagnosis: CHF
Comments: Note the lack of _a_ waves due to atrial fibrillation with normal respiratory variation.

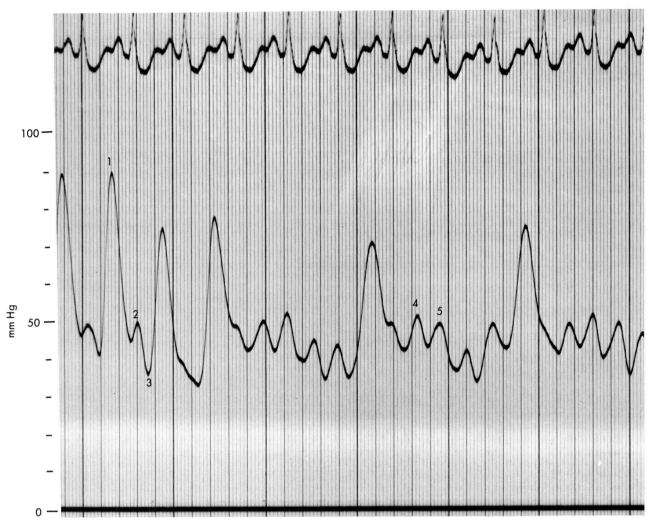

FIGURE 7-10

ANALYSIS

Rhythm:

Pressure(s):

Waveform characteristics and measurements:

1. _____ ; _____ mm Hg
2. _____ ; _____ mm Hg
3. _____ ; _____ mm Hg
4. _____ ; _____ mm Hg
5. _____ ; _____ mm Hg
6. _____ ; _____ mm Hg
7. _____ ; _____ mm Hg

Suspected abnormality/diagnosis:

Comments:

ANALYSIS of Figure 7-10

Rhythm: Sinus tachycardia

Pressure(s): PA/PAW

Waveform characteristics and measurements:

1.	PA systolic	; 85	mm Hg
2.	Dicrotic notch	;	mm Hg
3.	PA end-diastolic	; 38	mm Hg
4.	PAW *v* wave	; 48	mm Hg
5.	PAW *a* wave	; 49	mm Hg
6.		;	mm Hg
7.		;	mm Hg

Suspected abnormality/diagnosis: Pulmonary hypertension secondary to acute pulmonary edema

Comments: The first two beats are clearly a PA pressure. The following waveforms are mixed PA/PAW due to forward migration of the catheter tip. The pressure change from PA to PAW appears to be cyclical and regular, indicating that the changes follow the respiratory pattern. Slight withdrawal of the catheter tip should eliminate this problem.

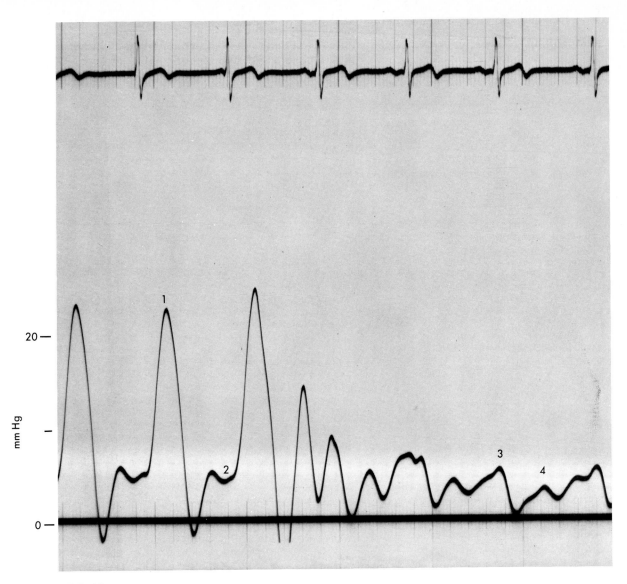

FIGURE 7-11

ANALYSIS

Rhythm:

Pressure(s):

Waveform characteristics and measurements:

1. _____ ; _____ mm Hg
2. _____ ; _____ mm Hg
3. _____ ; _____ mm Hg
4. _____ ; _____ mm Hg
5. _____ ; _____ mm Hg
6. _____ ; _____ mm Hg
7. _____ ; _____ mm Hg

Suspected abnormality/diagnosis:

Comments:

ANALYSIS of Figure 7-11

Rhythm: NSR

Pressure(s): RV to RA

Waveform characteristics and measurements:

#			value	units
1.	RV systolic	;	23	mm Hg
2.	RVedp	;	4	mm Hg
3.	RA *a* wave	;	6	mm Hg
4.	RA *v* wave	;	4	mm Hg
5.		;		mm Hg
6.		;		mm Hg
7.		;		mm Hg

Suspected abnormality/diagnosis: Catheter migration

Comments: The catheter tip has migrated backwards to the RV and on into the RA.

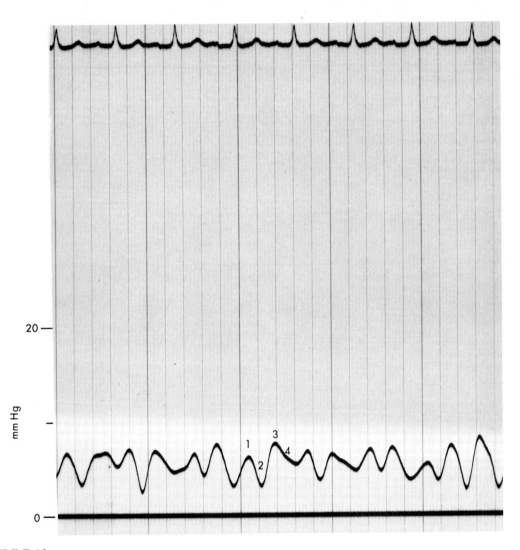

FIGURE 7-12

ANALYSIS

Rhythm:

Pressure(s):

Waveform characteristics and measurements:

1. _____ ; _____ mm Hg
2. _____ ; _____ mm Hg
3. _____ ; _____ mm Hg
4. _____ ; _____ mm Hg
5. _____ ; _____ mm Hg
6. _____ ; _____ mm Hg
7. _____ ; _____ mm Hg

Suspected abnormality/diagnosis:

Comments:

ANALYSIS of Figure 7-12

Rhythm: NSR
Pressure(s): PAW
Waveform characteristics and measurements:

#			
1.	_a_ Wave	7	mm Hg
2.	_x_ Descent		mm Hg
3.	_v_ Wave	7	mm Hg
4.	_y_ Descent		mm Hg
5.	Mean	5	mm Hg
6.			mm Hg
7.			mm Hg

Suspected abnormality/diagnosis: Normal PAW pressure
Comments:

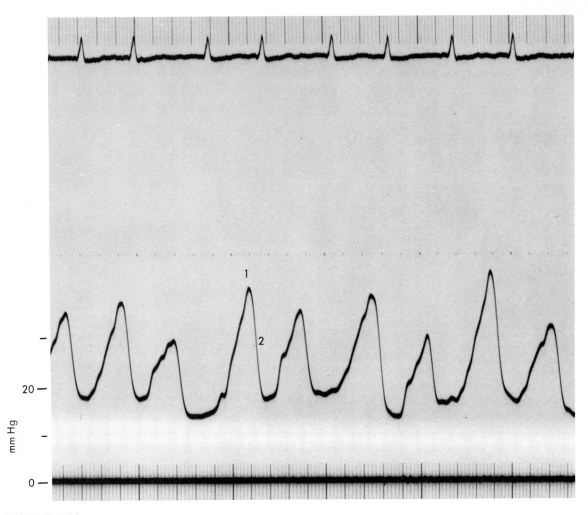

FIGURE 7-13

ANALYSIS

Rhythm:

Pressure(s):

Waveform characteristics and measurements:

1. _____ ; _____ mm Hg
2. _____ ; _____ mm Hg
3. _____ ; _____ mm Hg
4. _____ ; _____ mm Hg
5. _____ ; _____ mm Hg
6. _____ ; _____ mm Hg
7. _____ ; _____ mm Hg

Suspected abnormality/diagnosis:

Comments:

ANALYSIS of Figure 7-13

Rhythm: Atrial fibrillation

Pressure(s): PAW

Waveform characteristics and measurements:

1. _____ v Wave _____ ; _____ 37 _____ mm Hg
2. _____ y Descent _____ ; _____ mm Hg
3. _____ ; _____ mm Hg
4. _____ ; _____ mm Hg
5. _____ ; _____ mm Hg
6. _____ ; _____ mm Hg
7. _____ ; _____ mm Hg

Suspected abnormality/diagnosis: Mitral regurgitation

Comments: With atrial fibrillation and loss of electrical atrial systole there is a corresponding loss of mechanical atrial systole; therefore there are no a waves in this PAW waveform. There is only a v wave following each T wave. In this case the v wave is moderately elevated with a rapid y descent due to mitral regurgitation.

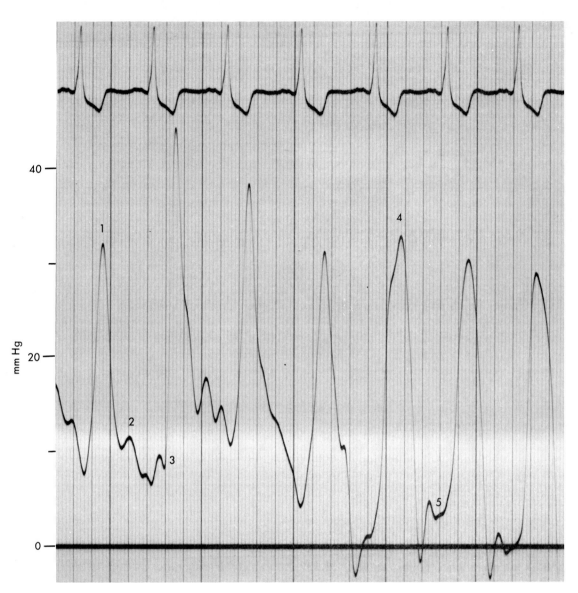

FIGURE 7-14

ANALYSIS

Rhythm:

Pressure(s):

Waveform characteristics and measurements:

1. _____ ; _____ mm Hg
2. _____ ; _____ mm Hg
3. _____ ; _____ mm Hg
4. _____ ; _____ mm Hg
5. _____ ; _____ mm Hg
6. _____ ; _____ mm Hg
7. _____ ; _____ mm Hg

Suspected abnormality/diagnosis:

Comments:

205

ANALYSIS   of Figure 7-14

Rhythm: NSR

Pressure(s): PA to RV

Waveform characteristics and measurements:

1.	PA systolic	;	35	mm Hg
2.	Dicrotic notch	;		mm Hg
3.	PA end-diastolic	;	10	mm Hg
4.	RV systolic	;	34	mm Hg
5.	RV end-diastolic	;	2	mm Hg
6.		;		mm Hg
7.		;		mm Hg

Suspected abnormality/diagnosis: Mild pulmonary hypertension with catheter migration

Comments: The catheter tip has slipped back from the PA to the RV. Note the similarity between the PA and RV systolic pressures and the discrepancy between the PA and RV diastolic pressures. If only the systolic digital value were being monitored in this patient, it would be possible to overlook the fact that the catheter tip has withdrawn back into the RV, a potentially hazardous situation. Monitoring the contour of the pressure waveform on the oscilloscope is essential to accurately identify the location of the pressure. Additionally, the digital mode selection should be set at *diastole* rather than *systole*, since it is that value which reflects the LVedp, and it is that value which will change immediately if the catheter tip falls into the RV. Balloon inflation is necessary to prevent ventricular dysrhythmias and allow flotation of the catheter tip back out to the PA.

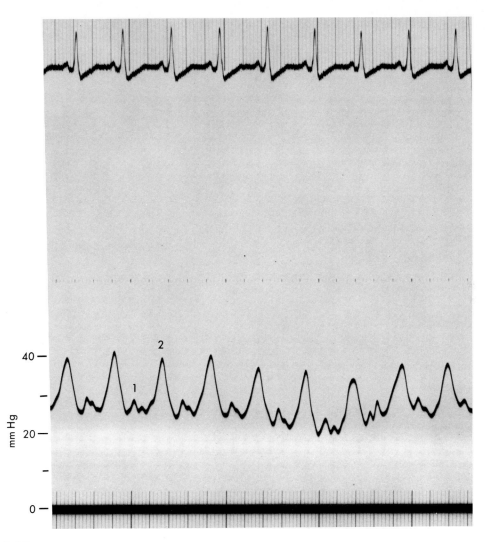

FIGURE 7-15

ANALYSIS

Rhythm:

Pressure(s):

Waveform characteristics and measurements:

1. _____ ; _____ mm Hg
2. _____ ; _____ mm Hg
3. _____ ; _____ mm Hg
4. _____ ; _____ mm Hg
5. _____ ; _____ mm Hg
6. _____ ; _____ mm Hg
7. _____ ; _____ mm Hg

Suspected abnormality/diagnosis:

Comments:

ANALYSIS of Figure 7-15

Rhythm: Sinus tachycardia

Pressure(s): PAW

Waveform characteristics and measurements:

1.	*a* Wave	;	27	mm Hg
2.	*v* Wave	;	38	mm Hg
3.		;		mm Hg
4.		;		mm Hg
5.		;		mm Hg
6.		;		mm Hg
7.		;		mm Hg

Suspected abnormality/diagnosis: LV failure with mitral regurgitation

Comments: The dominant and elevated *v* wave of 38 mm Hg suggests mild mitral regurgitation. The *a* wave of 25 mm Hg indicates LV failure. In this case the mitral regurgitation is secondary to LV failure with dilatation.

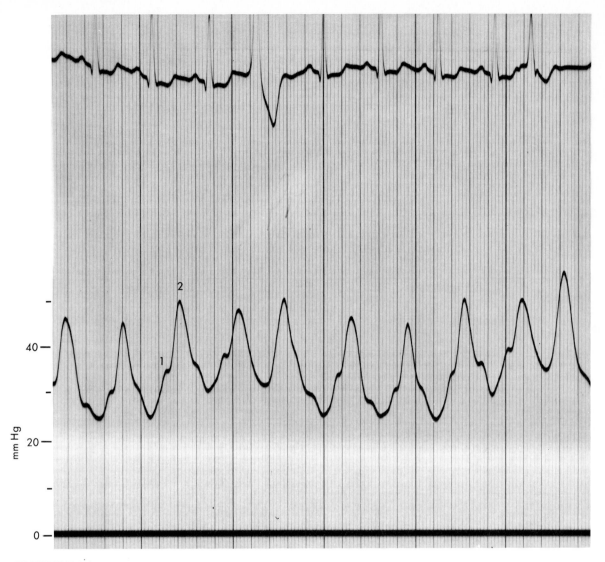

FIGURE 7-16

ANALYSIS

Rhythm:

Pressure(s):

Waveform characteristics and measurements:

1. _____ ; _____ mm Hg
2. _____ ; _____ mm Hg
3. _____ ; _____ mm Hg
4. _____ ; _____ mm Hg
5. _____ ; _____ mm Hg
6. _____ ; _____ mm Hg
7. _____ ; _____ mm Hg

Suspected abnormality/diagnosis:

Comments:

ANALYSIS of Figure 7-16

Rhythm: Sinus tachycardia with PVC and APC

Pressure(s): PAW

Waveform characteristics and measurements:

1.	*a* Wave	; 35	mm Hg
2.	*v* Wave	; 48	mm Hg
3.		;	mm Hg
4.		;	mm Hg
5.		;	mm Hg
6.		;	mm Hg
7.		;	mm Hg

Suspected abnormality/diagnosis: LV failure with mitral regurgitation

Comments: The early, dominant and elevated *v* wave of 48 mm Hg is due to mitral regurgitation; the *a* wave of 35 mm Hg indicates severe LV failure.

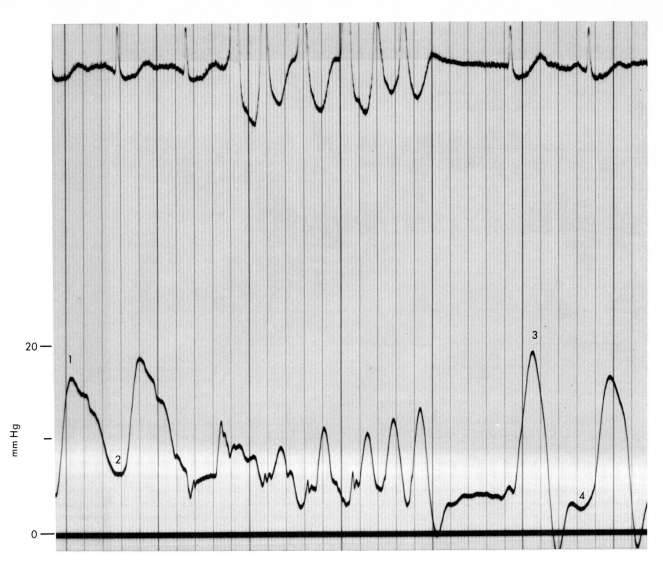

FIGURE 7-17

ANALYSIS

Rhythm:

Pressure(s):

Waveform characteristics and measurements:

1. _____ ; _____ mm Hg
2. _____ ; _____ mm Hg
3. _____ ; _____ mm Hg
4. _____ ; _____ mm Hg
5. _____ ; _____ mm Hg
6. _____ ; _____ mm Hg
7. _____ ; _____ mm Hg

Suspected abnormality/diagnosis:

Comments:

ANALYSIS of Figure 7-17

Rhythm: NSR with six-beat run of VT

Pressure(s): PA to RV

Waveform characteristics and measurements:

1.	PA systolic	;	19	mm Hg
2.	PA end-diastolic	;	7	mm Hg
3.	RV systolic	;	19	mm Hg
4.	RV end-diastolic	;	3	mm Hg
5.		;		mm Hg
6.		;		mm Hg
7.		;		mm Hg

Suspected abnormality/diagnosis: Normal

Comments: The catheter tip has fallen from the PA into the RV, causing a brief run of VT. Repositioning of the catheter is necessary to prevent the occurrence of further ventricular arrhythmias. Note the similarity between the PA and RV systolic pressures but the disparity in the diastolic values with the RV diastolic pressure falling below baseline.

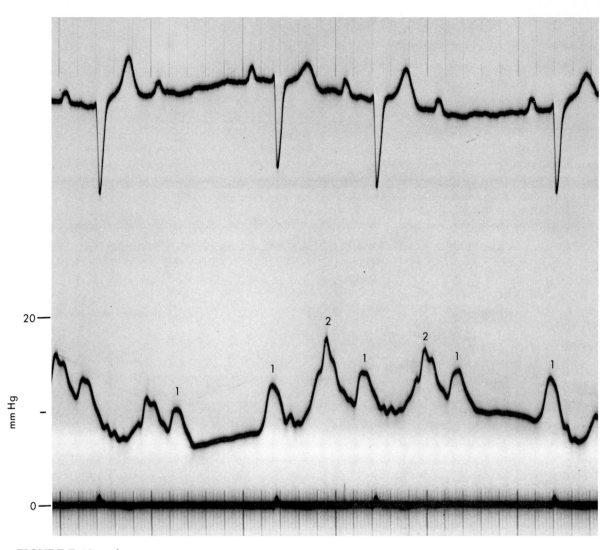

FIGURE 7-18

ANALYSIS

Rhythm:

Pressure(s):

Waveform characteristics and measurements:

1. _____ ; _____ mm Hg
2. _____ ; _____ mm Hg
3. _____ ; _____ mm Hg
4. _____ ; _____ mm Hg
5. _____ ; _____ mm Hg
6. _____ ; _____ mm Hg
7. _____ ; _____ mm Hg

Suspected abnormality/diagnosis:

Comments:

ANALYSIS of Figure 7-18

Rhythm: Second-degree AV block with Wenckebach phenomenon

Pressure(s): PAW

Waveform characteristics and measurements:

1.	*a* Wave	;	14	mm Hg
2.	*v* Wave	;	16	mm Hg
3.	Mean	;	12	mm Hg
4.		;		mm Hg
5.		;		mm Hg
6.		;		mm Hg
7.		;		mm Hg

Suspected abnormality/diagnosis: Mild CHF

Comments: Each atrial depolarization (P wave) is followed by atrial systole (PAW *a* wave). However, since every third impulse is not conducted, a *v* wave does not follow each *a* wave. Careful analysis of this tracing shows PAW *a* waves following each ECG P wave and a *v* wave after each ventricular depolarization, albeit at a different rate.

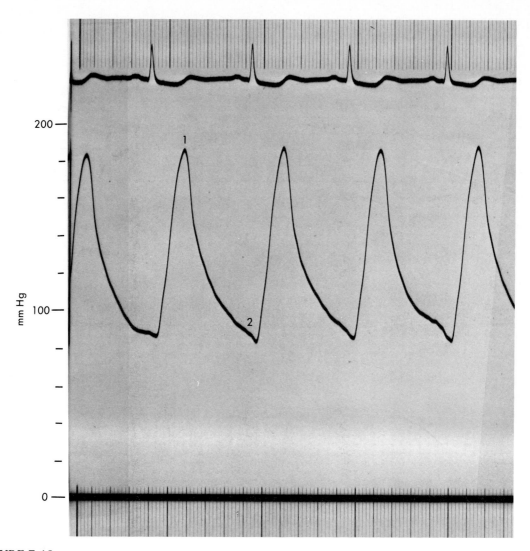

FIGURE 7-19

ANALYSIS

Rhythm:

Pressure(s):

Waveform characteristics and measurements:

1. _____ ; _____ mm Hg
2. _____ ; _____ mm Hg
3. _____ ; _____ mm Hg
4. _____ ; _____ mm Hg
5. _____ ; _____ mm Hg
6. _____ ; _____ mm Hg
7. _____ ; _____ mm Hg

Suspected abnormality/diagnosis:

Comments:

ANALYSIS of Figure 7-19

Rhythm: NSR

Pressure(s): Radial artery

Waveform characteristics and measurements:

1.	Arterial systolic	; 180	mm Hg
2.	Arterial end-diastolic	; 85	mm Hg
3.		;	mm Hg
4.		;	mm Hg
5.		;	mm Hg
6.		;	mm Hg
7.		;	mm Hg

Suspected abnormality/diagnosis: Aortic regurgitation

Comments: Note the wide pulse pressure (95 mm Hg) and absent dicrotic notch, which are indicative of aortic regurgitation.

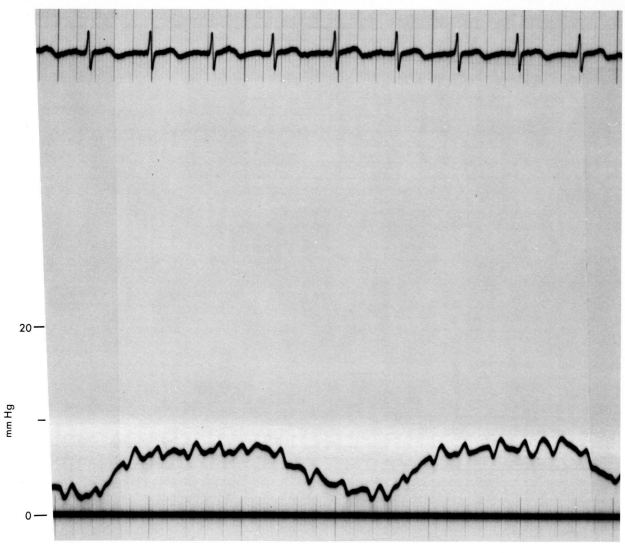

FIGURE 7-20

ANALYSIS

Rhythm:

Pressure(s):

Waveform characteristics and measurements:

1. _____ ; _____ mm Hg
2. _____ ; _____ mm Hg
3. _____ ; _____ mm Hg
4. _____ ; _____ mm Hg
5. _____ ; _____ mm Hg
6. _____ ; _____ mm Hg
7. _____ ; _____ mm Hg

Suspected abnormality/diagnosis:

Comments:

ANALYSIS of Figure 7-20

Rhythm: Regular supraventricular tachycardia

Pressure(s): PAW

Waveform characteristics and measurements:

1.	Mean	;	6	mm Hg
2.		;		mm Hg
3.		;		mm Hg
4.		;		mm Hg
5.		;		mm Hg
6.		;		mm Hg
7.		;		mm Hg

Suspected abnormality/diagnosis: Hypovolemia

Comments: Note the normal respiratory variation in this low PAW pressure.

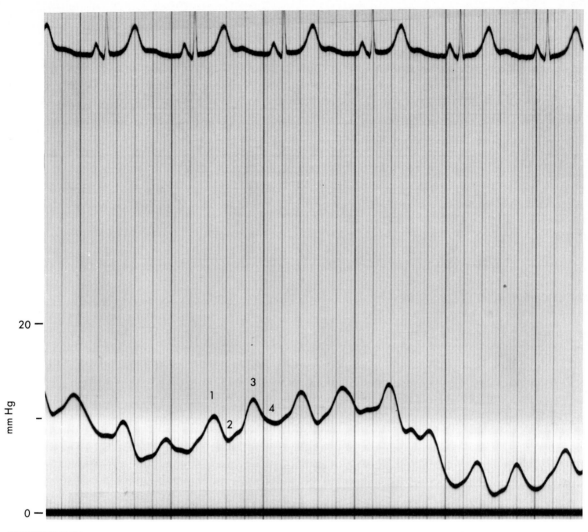

FIGURE 7-21

ANALYSIS

Rhythm:

Pressure(s):

Waveform characteristics and measurements:

1. _____ ; _____ mm Hg
2. _____ ; _____ mm Hg
3. _____ ; _____ mm Hg
4. _____ ; _____ mm Hg
5. _____ ; _____ mm Hg
6. _____ ; _____ mm Hg
7. _____ ; _____ mm Hg

Suspected abnormality/diagnosis:

Comments:

ANALYSIS of Figure 7-21

Rhythm: NSR

Pressure(s): PAW

Waveform characteristics and measurements:

1.	*a* Wave	; 12	mm Hg
2.	*x* Descent	;	mm Hg
3.	*v* Wave	; 13	mm Hg
4.	*y* Descent	;	mm Hg
5.	Mean	; 11	mm Hg
6.		;	mm Hg
7.		;	mm Hg

Suspected abnormality/diagnosis: Normal PAW pressure

Comments:

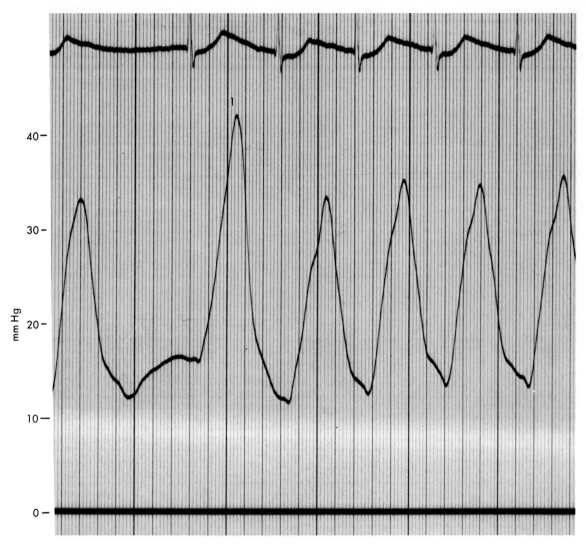

FIGURE 7-22

ANALYSIS

Rhythm:

Pressure(s):

Waveform characteristics and measurements:

1. _____ ; _____ mm Hg
2. _____ ; _____ mm Hg
3. _____ ; _____ mm Hg
4. _____ ; _____ mm Hg
5. _____ ; _____ mm Hg
6. _____ ; _____ mm Hg
7. _____ ; _____ mm Hg

Suspected abnormality/diagnosis:

Comments:

ANALYSIS of Figure 7-22

Rhythm: Nodal

Pressure(s): PAW

Waveform characteristics and measurements:

1. _____ v Wave _____ ; _____ 35 _____ mm Hg
2. _____ ; _____ mm Hg
3. _____ ; _____ mm Hg
4. _____ ; _____ mm Hg
5. _____ ; _____ mm Hg
6. _____ ; _____ mm Hg
7. _____ ; _____ mm Hg

Suspected abnormality/diagnosis: Severe mitral regurgitation

Comments: This PAW waveform has an unusual appearance because of the lack of a waves and the early appearance of the elevated v waves. Note the increase in the size of the v wave (reflecting an increased regurgitant volume) following a prolonged RR interval.

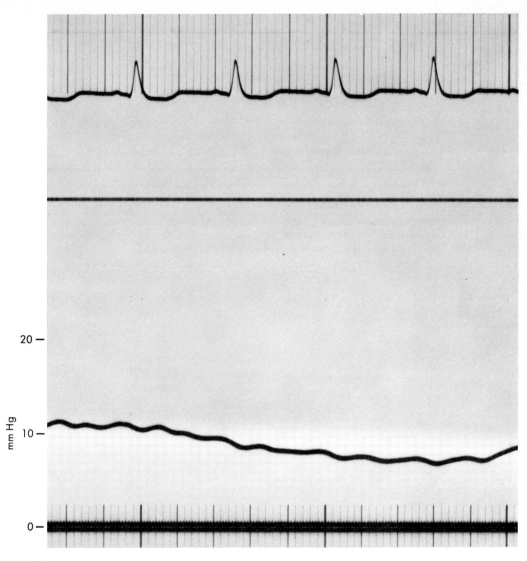

FIGURE 7-23

ANALYSIS

Rhythm:

Pressure(s):

Waveform characteristics and measurements:

1. _____ ; _____ mm Hg
2. _____ ; _____ mm Hg
3. _____ ; _____ mm Hg
4. _____ ; _____ mm Hg
5. _____ ; _____ mm Hg
6. _____ ; _____ mm Hg
7. _____ ; _____ mm Hg

Suspected abnormality/diagnosis:

Comments:

ANALYSIS of Figure 7-23

Rhythm: NSR

Pressure(s): Unknown

Waveform characteristics and measurements:

1. _____ ; _____ mm Hg
2. _____ ; _____ mm Hg
3. _____ ; _____ mm Hg
4. _____ ; _____ mm Hg
5. _____ ; _____ mm Hg
6. _____ ; _____ mm Hg
7. _____ ; _____ mm Hg

Suspected abnormality/diagnosis:

Comments: This very damped pressure is unidentifiable and inaccurate. After deflation of the balloon to ensure that it is not wedged, the catheter should be aspirated and flushed.

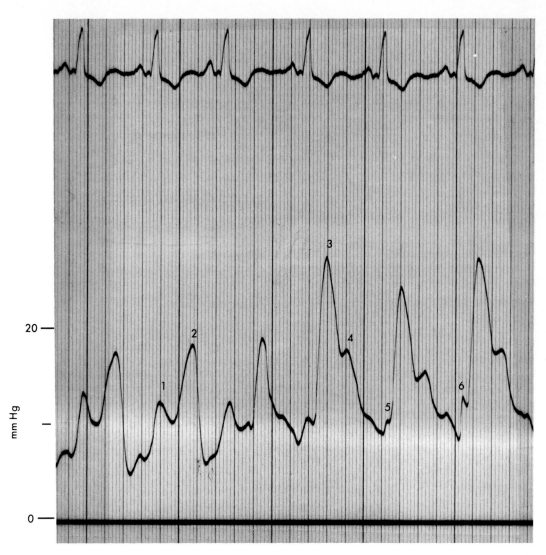

FIGURE 7-24

ANALYSIS

Rhythm:

Pressure(s):

Waveform characteristics and measurements:

1. _____ ; _____ mm Hg
2. _____ ; _____ mm Hg
3. _____ ; _____ mm Hg
4. _____ ; _____ mm Hg
5. _____ ; _____ mm Hg
6. _____ ; _____ mm Hg
7. _____ ; _____ mm Hg

Suspected abnormality/diagnosis:

Comments:

ANALYSIS of Figure 7-24

Rhythm: NSR

Pressure(s): PAW to PA

Waveform characteristics and measurements:

1.	PAW *a* wave	;	12	mm Hg
2.	PAW *v* wave	;	19	mm Hg
3.	PA systolic	;	28	mm Hg
4.	Dicrotic notch	;		mm Hg
5.	PA end-diastolic	;	11	mm Hg
6.	*a* Wave	;	11	mm Hg
7.		;		mm Hg

Suspected abnormality/diagnosis: Mild LV failure with mild mitral regurgitation

Comments: The somewhat dominant and elevated PAW *v* wave of 19 mm Hg suggests mild regurgitation of blood through the mitral valve during systole. The rapid *y* descent is another indication of mitral regurgitation and is due to the enhanced emptying of the LA through the mitral valve. The slight elevation of the PAW *a* wave (12 mm Hg) indicates very mild LV failure. The waveform labeled 6 may be the *a* wave of the PAW reflected back in the PA pressure waveform. Note its correlation to the P wave of the ECG and the PAW *a* wave.

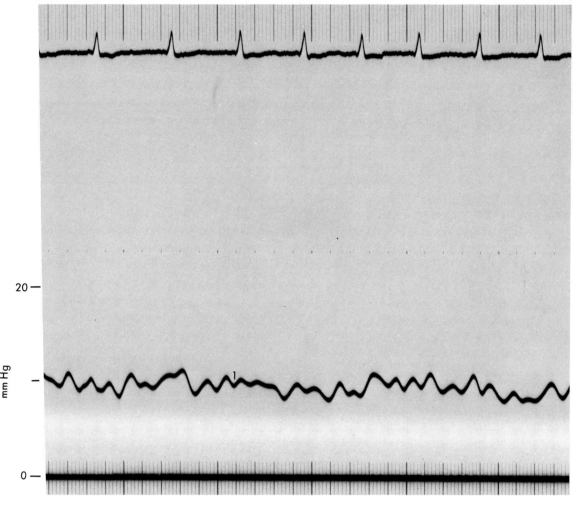

FIGURE 7-25

ANALYSIS

Rhythm:

Pressure(s):

Waveform characteristics and measurements:

1. _____	;	_____ mm Hg
2. _____	;	_____ mm Hg
3. _____	;	_____ mm Hg
4. _____	;	_____ mm Hg
5. _____	;	_____ mm Hg
6. _____	;	_____ mm Hg
7. _____	;	_____ mm Hg

Suspected abnormality/diagnosis:

Comments:

ANALYSIS of Figure 7-25

Rhythm: Atrial fibrillation

Pressure(s): RA

Waveform characteristics and measurements:

1.	Fibrillatory waves	;	____ mm Hg
2.	Mean	;	10 mm Hg
3.	____	;	____ mm Hg
4.	____	;	____ mm Hg
5.	____	;	____ mm Hg
6.	____	;	____ mm Hg
7.	____	;	____ mm Hg

Suspected abnormality/diagnosis: Mild right heart failure

Comments: With atrial fibrillation and a lack of atrial systole, we can expect to see only a v wave for each T wave. The numerous small pressure waves reflect fibrillatory activity of the atrium. Identification of the v wave is difficult but is hemodynamically insignificant, since all pressure fluctuations are essentially equal, resulting in a mean RA pressure of approximately 10 mm Hg, which is somewhat elevated.

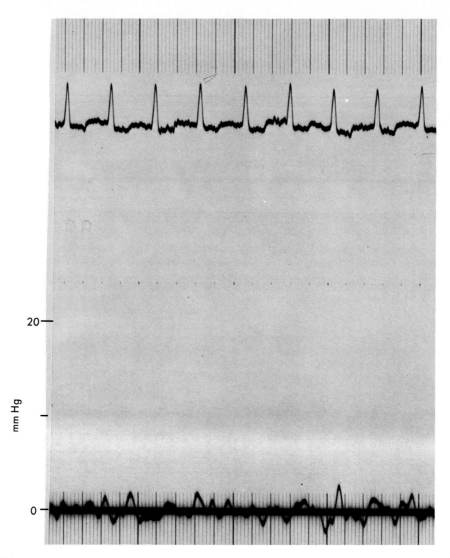

FIGURE 7-26

ANALYSIS

Rhythm:

Pressure(s):

Waveform characteristics and measurements:

1. _____ ; _____ mm Hg
2. _____ ; _____ mm Hg
3. _____ ; _____ mm Hg
4. _____ ; _____ mm Hg
5. _____ ; _____ mm Hg
6. _____ ; _____ mm Hg
7. _____ ; _____ mm Hg

Suspected abnormality/diagnosis:

Comments:

229

ANALYSIS of Figure 7-26

Rhythm: NSR

Pressure(s): RA

Waveform characteristics and measurements:

1. _____ Mean _____ ; ____0____ mm Hg
2. _____ ; _____ mm Hg
3. _____ ; _____ mm Hg
4. _____ ; _____ mm Hg
5. _____ ; _____ mm Hg
6. _____ ; _____ mm Hg
7. _____ ; _____ mm Hg

Suspected abnormality/diagnosis: Inaccurate pressure

Comments: This pressure waveform is abnormally low due to incorrect placement of the transducer air reference above the level of the right atrium.

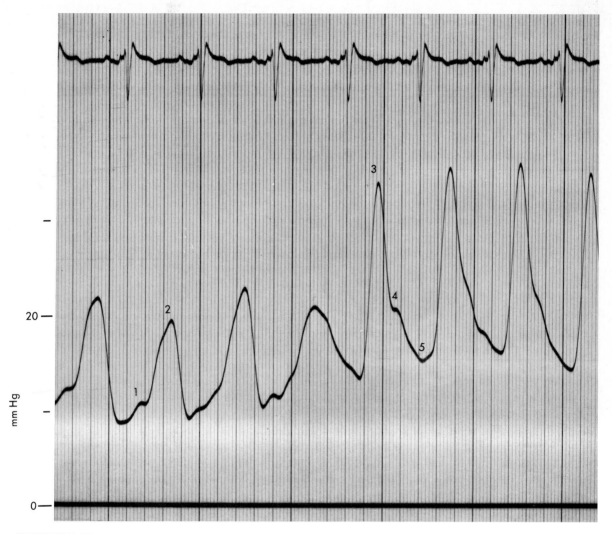

FIGURE 7-27

ANALYSIS

Rhythm:

Pressure(s):

Waveform characteristics and measurements:

1. _____ ; _____ mm Hg
2. _____ ; _____ mm Hg
3. _____ ; _____ mm Hg
4. _____ ; _____ mm Hg
5. _____ ; _____ mm Hg
6. _____ ; _____ mm Hg
7. _____ ; _____ mm Hg

Suspected abnormality/diagnosis:

Comments:

ANALYSIS   of Figure 7-27

Rhythm: NSR

Pressure(s): PAW to PA

Waveform characteristics and measurements:

1.	PAW *a* wave	;	12	mm Hg
2.	PAW *v* wave	;	22	mm Hg
3.	PA systolic	;	35	mm Hg
4.	Dicrotic notch	;		mm Hg
5.	PA end-diastolic	;	14	mm Hg
6.		;		mm Hg
7.		;		mm Hg

Suspected abnormality/diagnosis: Mitral regurgitation

Comments: The dominant and elevated PAW *v* wave and rapid *y* descent indicate mitral regurgitation with an increase in LA volume during ventricular systole. The PAW *a* wave is of high normal value. Note the correlation between the PAW *a* wave (12 mm Hg) and the PAedp (14 mm Hg).

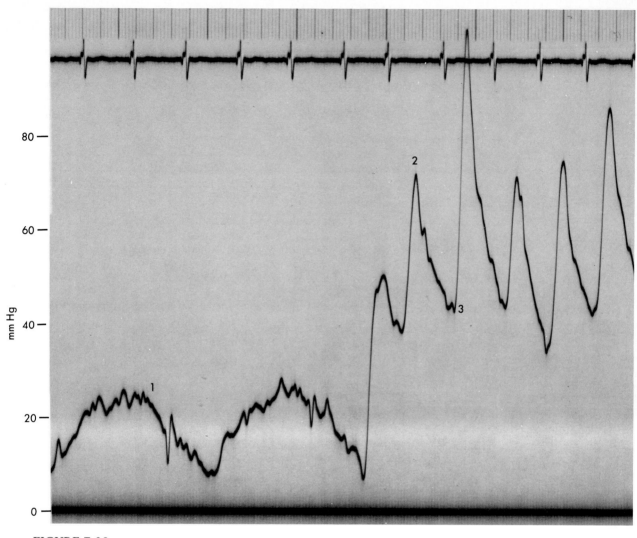

FIGURE 7-28

ANALYSIS

Rhythm:

Pressure(s):

Waveform characteristics and measurements:

1. _____ ; _____ mm Hg
2. _____ ; _____ mm Hg
3. _____ ; _____ mm Hg
4. _____ ; _____ mm Hg
5. _____ ; _____ mm Hg
6. _____ ; _____ mm Hg
7. _____ ; _____ mm Hg

Suspected abnormality/diagnosis:

Comments:

ANALYSIS of Figure 7-28

Rhythm: Atrial fibrillation

Pressure(s): PAW to PA

Waveform characteristics and measurements:

1.	PAW mean	;	16	mm Hg
2.	PA systolic	;	78	mm Hg
3.	PA end-diastolic	;	40	mm Hg
4.		;		mm Hg
5.		;		mm Hg
6.		;		mm Hg
7.		;		mm Hg

Suspected abnormality/diagnosis: Primary pulmonary hypertension

Comments: The rapid ventricular rate, the marked respiratory variation, and the fibrillatory waves in the PAW pressure make identification of the v wave difficult. For this reason the mean PAW pressure is used to reflect LVedp. Note the marked disparity between the PAW mean pressure (16 mm Hg) and the PAedp (40 mm Hg). This is due to primary pulmonary vascular disease and elevated PVR. In this situation only the PAW pressure can be used as a reflection of LVedp.

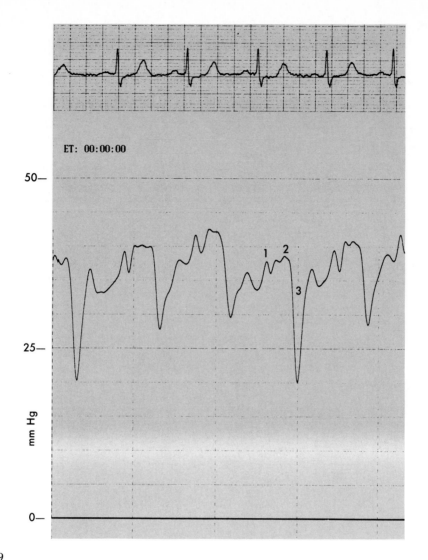

ET: 00:00:00

FIGURE 7-29

ANALYSIS

Rhythm:

Pressure(s):

Waveform characteristics and measurements:

1. _____ ; _____ mm Hg
2. _____ ; _____ mm Hg
3. _____ ; _____ mm Hg
4. _____ ; _____ mm Hg
5. _____ ; _____ mm Hg
6. _____ ; _____ mm Hg
7. _____ ; _____ mm Hg

Suspected abnormality/diagnosis:

Comments:

ANALYSIS of Figure 7-29

Rhythm: NSR

Pressure(s): RA

Waveform characteristics and measurements:

1.	*a* Wave	; 39	mm Hg
2.	*v* Wave	; 40	mm Hg
3.	*y* Descent	;	mm Hg
4.	Mean	; 37	mm Hg
5.		;	mm Hg
6.		;	mm Hg
7.		;	mm Hg

Suspected abnormality/diagnosis: Constrictive pericarditis

Comments: The elevated *a* and *v* waves with a very brief *x* descent following the *a* wave, and an exaggerated *y* descent after the *v* wave are typical findings in constrictive pericarditis.

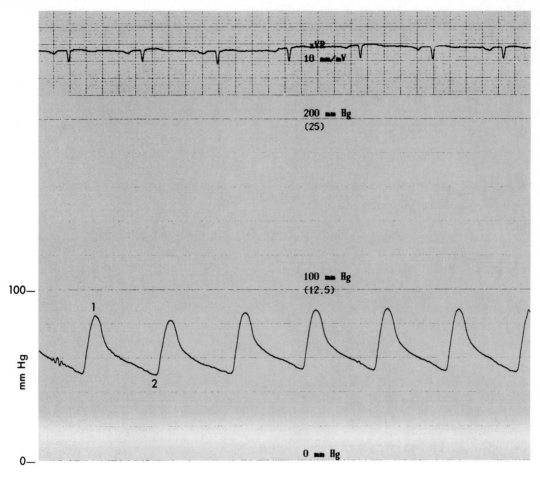

FIGURE 7-30

ANALYSIS

Rhythm:

Pressure(s):

Waveform characteristics and measurements:

1. _____ ; _____ mm Hg
2. _____ ; _____ mm Hg
3. _____ ; _____ mm Hg
4. _____ ; _____ mm Hg
5. _____ ; _____ mm Hg
6. _____ ; _____ mm Hg
7. _____ ; _____ mm Hg

Suspected abnormality/diagnosis:

Comments:

ANALYSIS of Figure 7-30

Rhythm: NSR

Pressure(s): Radial artery

Waveform characteristics and measurements:

1.	Systolic	;	84	mm Hg
2.	Diastolic	;	50	mm Hg
3.		;		mm Hg
4.		;		mm Hg
5.		;		mm Hg
6.		;		mm Hg
7.		;		mm Hg

Suspected abnormality/diagnosis: Hypotension

Comments: The low systolic and pulse pressure of this arterial waveform are due to low stroke volume. A diastolic arterial pressure of 50 mm Hg seriously jeopardizes coronary blood flow.

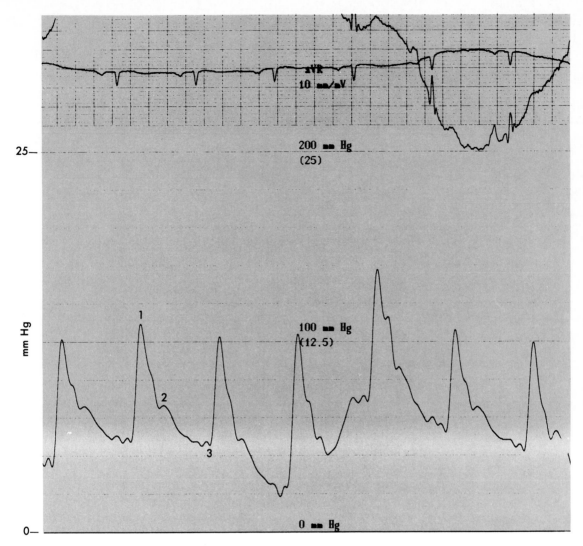

FIGURE 7-31

ANALYSIS

Rhythm:

Pressure(s):

Waveform characteristics and measurements:

1. _____	;	_____ mm Hg
2. _____	;	_____ mm Hg
3. _____	;	_____ mm Hg
4. _____	;	_____ mm Hg
5. _____	;	_____ mm Hg
6. _____	;	_____ mm Hg
7. _____	;	_____ mm Hg

Suspected abnormality/diagnosis:

Comments:

ANALYSIS of Figure 7-31

Rhythm: NSR

Pressure(s): PA

Waveform characteristics and measurements:

1.	Systolic	;	1-3	mm Hg
2.	Dicrotic notch	;		mm Hg
3.	Diastolic	;	5	mm Hg
4.		;		mm Hg
5.		;		mm Hg
6.		;		mm Hg
7.		;		mm Hg

Suspected abnormality/diagnosis: Hypovolemia

Comments: This very low PA pressure reflects diminished volume ejected from the right heart. Such a finding can often be seen in patients with RV infarction in whom output from the right heart is very low.

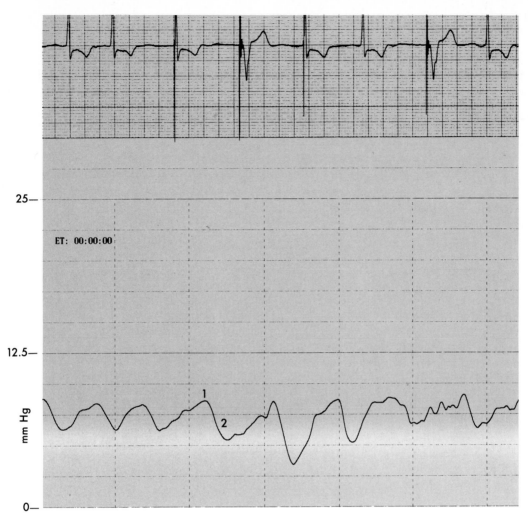

FIGURE 7-32

ANALYSIS

Rhythm:

Pressure(s):

Waveform characteristics and measurements:

1.	;	mm Hg
2.	;	mm Hg
3.	;	mm Hg
4.	;	mm Hg
5.	;	mm Hg
6.	;	mm Hg
7.	;	mm Hg

Suspected abnormality/diagnosis:

Comments:

ANALYSIS of Figure 7-32

Rhythm: Atrial fibrillation with VVI pacemaker
Pressure(s): RA
Waveform characteristics and measurements:

1.	_v_ Wave	; 8	mm Hg
2.	Mean	; 6	mm Hg
3.		;	mm Hg
4.		;	mm Hg
5.		;	mm Hg
6.		;	mm Hg
7.		;	mm Hg

Suspected abnormality/diagnosis: Normal RA pressure
Comments:

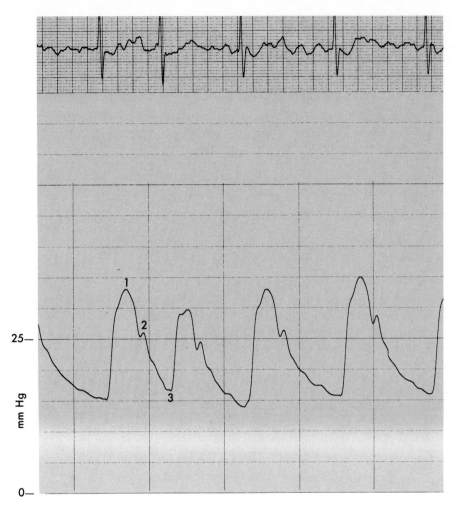

FIGURE 7-33

ANALYSIS

Rhythm:

Pressure(s):

Waveform characteristics and measurements:

1. _____ ; _____ mm Hg
2. _____ ; _____ mm Hg
3. _____ ; _____ mm Hg
4. _____ ; _____ mm Hg
5. _____ ; _____ mm Hg
6. _____ ; _____ mm Hg
7. _____ ; _____ mm Hg

Suspected abnormality/diagnosis:

Comments:

ANALYSIS of Figure 7-33

Rhythm: Atrial fibrillation/flutter

Pressure(s): PA

Waveform characteristics and measurements:

1.	Systolic	; 32	mm Hg
2.	Dicrotic notch	;	mm Hg
3.	Diastolic	; 15	mm Hg
4.		;	mm Hg
5.		;	mm Hg
6.		;	mm Hg
7.		;	mm Hg

Suspected abnormality/diagnosis: Mild pulmonary hypertension

Comments: This PA pressure is mildly elevated with changes in the systolic value associated with changes in the RR intervals.

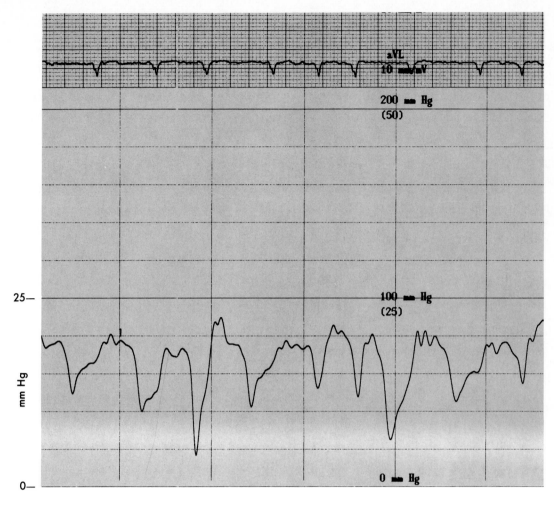

aVL
10 mm/mV

200 mm Hg
(50)

25—

100 mm Hg
(25)

mm Hg

0— 0 mm Hg

FIGURE 7-34

ANALYSIS

Rhythm:

Pressure(s):

Waveform characteristics and measurements:

1. _____ ; _____ mm Hg
2. _____ ; _____ mm Hg
3. _____ ; _____ mm Hg
4. _____ ; _____ mm Hg
5. _____ ; _____ mm Hg
6. _____ ; _____ mm Hg
7. _____ ; _____ mm Hg

Suspected abnormality/diagnosis:

Comments:

ANALYSIS of Figure 7-34

Rhythm: Atrial fibrillation

Pressure(s): RA

Waveform characteristics and measurements:

1.	*v* Wave	;	20	mm Hg
2.	Mean	;	17	mm Hg
3.		;		mm Hg
4.		;		mm Hg
5.		;		mm Hg
6.		;		mm Hg
7.		;		mm Hg

Suspected abnormality/diagnosis: RV failure with tricuspid regurgitation

Comments: The *v* wave of this RA pressure is elevated, as is the overall mean pressure. This is due to RV failure with associated tricuspid regurgitation.

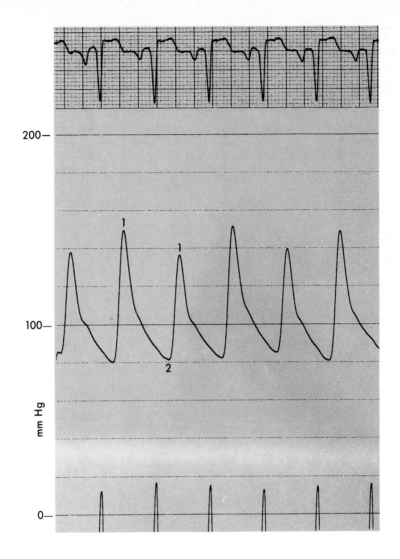

FIGURE 7-35

ANALYSIS

Rhythm:

Pressure(s):

Waveform characteristics and measurements:

1. _____ ; _____ mm Hg
2. _____ ; _____ mm Hg
3. _____ ; _____ mm Hg
4. _____ ; _____ mm Hg
5. _____ ; _____ mm Hg
6. _____ ; _____ mm Hg
7. _____ ; _____ mm Hg

Suspected abnormality/diagnosis:

Comments:

ANALYSIS   of Figure 7-35

Rhythm: NSR

Pressure(s): Femoral artery

Waveform characteristics and measurements:

1.	Systolic	;	128-144	mm Hg
2.	Diastolic	;	80	mm Hg
3.		;		mm Hg
4.		;		mm Hg
5.		;		mm Hg
6.		;		mm Hg
7.		;		mm Hg

Suspected abnormality/diagnosis: LV failure

Comments: The presence of pulsus alternans is apparent in this arterial waveform and is due to severe LV failure. The poorly defined dicrotic notch is a normal phenomenon in the femoral artery pressure wave.

Bibliography

Alpert JS: Hemodynamic monitoring: the basics, Primary Cardiol, pp 113-126, May 1981.

Daily EK and Schroeder JS: Techniques in bedside hemodynamic monitoring, ed 4, St Louis, 1989, The CV Mosby Co.

Forrester JS, Diamond G, and Swan HJ: Bedside diagnosis of latent cardiac complications in acutely ill patients, JAMA 226:60-61, 1973.

Gorlin R: Practical cardiac hemodynamics, N Engl J Med 296:203-205, 1977.

Grossman W: Cardiac catheterization and angiography, Philadelphia, 1980, Lea & Febiger.

Hancock EW: On the elastic and rigid forms of constrictive pericarditis, Am Heart J 100:917-923, 1980.

Kelman GR: Applied cardiovascular physiology, Boston, 1979, Butterworths Inc.

King ED: Influence of mechanical ventilation and pulmonary disease on pulmonary artery pressure monitoring, CMAJ 121:901-904, 1979.

Lorell M: Right ventricular infarction: clinical diagnosis and differentiation from cardiac tamponade and pericardial constriction, Am J Cardiol 43:465-471, 1979.

Sharkey SW: Beyond the wedge: clinical physiology and the Swan-Ganz catheter, Am J Med 83:111-122, 1987.

Understanding hemodynamic measurements made with the Swan-Ganz catheter, Santa Ana, Calif, 1979, Edwards Laboratories.

Slide Series

This slide series includes all the hemodynamic waveforms presented in this book. Each slide is numbered and coded according to the corresponding figure number in this book.

Ideal for in-service education, symposiums, and seminars, this series is also valuable for self-instruction when accompanied by this text.

The entire series of slides can be purchased for $210.00. To order, copy and fill in the order form below and mail with a check or money order to:

Daily and Schroeder
Falk Cardiovascular Research Building
Stanford University Medical Center
Stanford, CA 94305

- -

Please send me one teaching slide series of hemodynamic waveforms from *Hemodynamic Waveforms: Exercises in Interpretation and Analysis,* ed 2, by EK Daily and JS Schroeder, St. Louis, 1990. The CV Mosby Co.

Name _____

Street _____

City _____ State _____ Zip _____

One slide series $210.00

California residents, add $15.75 (7½% tax)   _____

Canadians, add $25 if paid in Canadian currency   _____

Overseas mailing, add $10   _____

Enclosed is a check or money order for   _____ (TOTAL)

Get a new *focus* on critical care nursing

If you're committed to continuing your personal and professional growth in critical care nursing, you'll want to become a regular reader of FOCUS ON CRITICAL CARE.

Six times a year, FOCUS brings you *highly relevant* clinical information targeting today's most important topics in critical care. Moreover, the Journal gives you an insightful look at the larger issues facing nurses, serving as a forum for the ideas and personal experiences of your nursing colleagues.

FOCUS has a 4-color, magazine format that makes it easy and enjoyable to read. The tables and charts within articles provide you with key information quickly and concisely.

All articles in FOCUS ON CRITICAL CARE are original, peer-reviewed contributions. Recent topics have included:

- Emergency-department overcrowding: Meeting the crisis with new creativity
- A nursing perspective on the use of unlicensed personnel
- Individual actions to improve nursing's image
- An instructor's return to clinical nursing: Can you go home again?
- Writing for a nursing journal
- Overtime: A professional responsibility?
- Acute crack cocaine intoxication: A case study
- Family member perceptions of a cardiac surgery event
- Privacy issues in AIDS testing and treatment

In addition, regular departments in FOCUS address legal issues in nursing, research reviews (and implications for practice), software and book reviews, educational opportunities, and news from the American Association of Critical-Care Nurses, for which FOCUS is an official journal.

Don't miss another issue of FOCUS ON CRITICAL CARE. Let us hear from you today!

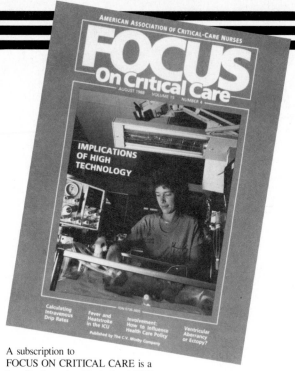

A subscription to
FOCUS ON CRITICAL CARE is a
benefit of membership in the AACN.

**To begin your subscription, simply call
Mosby-Year Book toll-free: 1-800-325-4177, ext. 7351.**

Outside the U.S., call (314) 872-8370, ext. 7351.
Fax: 314-432-1380.

Or write:
Mosby-Year Book, Journal Circulation Department,
11830 Westline Industrial Dr., St. Louis, MO 63146 U.S.A.

FOCUS ON CRITICAL CARE.
(Bimonthly; six issues per year)

1990 Annual Rates	U.S.	International
Individual	$21.00	$27.00
Student (full-time)	13.00	19.00
Institutional	54.00	60.00

Individual and student subscriptions must be in the name of, billed to, and paid for by the individual.

Please allow 6-8 weeks for processing your order.

Price of international subscriptions includes surface-mail postage. Contact Publisher for airmail rates if faster delivery is required.   J2240AZZ